FIT TO BE 50

FIT TO BE 50

Samantha Lee

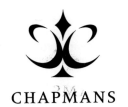

CHAPMANS

For Haydn and Pearl,
who've been fifty for the last twenty years!

Chapmans Publishers Ltd
141–143 Drury Lane
London WC2B 5TB

A CIP catalogue record for this book is available from the British Library

ISBN 1-85592-586-9

First published by Chapmans 1992
Copyright © 1992 by Samantha Lee

The right of Samantha Lee to be identified as the author of this work has been asserted by her in accordance with the Copyright, Designs and Patents Act 1988.

Design by
Sue Clarke

Exercise diagrams by
Coral Mula

Photoset by
M.C. Typeset Limited, Rochester, Kent.

Printed and bound in Great Britain by
Butler & Tanner Ltd, Frome and London

'Regular exercise and physical activity may be the closest thing we have to that long sought after Fountain of Youth.'

Len Kravitz and Craig J. Cisar, *Idea Today*, January 1991.

ACKNOWLEDGEMENTS

My sincere and heartfelt thanks to my agents Diana Tyler and Ruth Needham, for their unfailing efforts on my behalf. To Marjory and Ian Chapman for taking a chance on an unknown, and my editors Pam Dix and Yvonne Holland for all their help and advice. To Jack and Charlie for lending me their flat in Malaga to block out the rough draft. To Brent, Jane and Darryl at Fitness Professionals and Dorothy Dobson at Dundee University who added impetus and inspiration. To Dee Taylor who, quite literally, changed my life, and to Moira Holden, Top Gun at the Aberdeen Petroleum Club, and true friend. To all my wonderful 'chaps' who, over the years, have kept my classes full of life and my life full of laughter. To everybody who agreed to be quoted or paraphrased in this book. And last but not least to Pete and Stevie, for putting up with me.

CONTENTS

DISCLAIMER

The exercises in this book are aimed at men and women of average health and fitness. Anyone with back problems, a pre-existing medical condition or who has recently undergone an operation, should get their doctor's clearance before undertaking any exercise regime.

PROLOGUE

This is a book about getting fit at fifty. It is not a magic wand. It will not work by osmosis. There is enough information in the following pages to change your life, your shape, your attitudes and your future – for the better. But only if you *act* on it.

As Einstein said: 'Knowledge is experience – everything else is just information.'

To get results you will need to invest half an hour a day – six days a week – in this enterprise: half an hour – that's all, and one day off for good behaviour.

If you cannot find half an hour anywhere else, you will have to give up watching *The Nine O'clock News*. Considering some of the news these days, this will probably make you feel considerably better almost immediately. And feeling better is what being fit, at any age, is all about.

Fifty is a *great* age. You are mature enough to come to terms with yourself, young enough to benefit from the experience. And whereas, until quite recently it was believed that after a certain point you should take it easy for fear of wearing yourself out, current research shows that it is *inactivity* which causes the systems to break down, the bones to soften, the muscles to atrophy. A good example of this is the individual (of whatever age) who breaks a leg. After a couple of months of sedentary living the plaster is removed to reveal a limb, wasted and withered from lack of use. The patient then has to undergo physio-therapy and a pretty rigorous training routine to bring it back in line with its active twin.

Exactly the same principle applies to the body in general. Use it – if you don't want to lose it. It is *underuse*, the kind brought on by other people's attitudes towards the capabilities of anyone over fifty, that causes physical decline. This decline is totally unnecessary, because muscle doesn't even begin to lose its capacity to change and grow until after the milestone three-score years and ten has passed. Up until that point you can actually improve your physical condition. After that you can, at the very least, preserve the status quo.

So the good news is that you don't have to fall apart at the seams. The bad news is that it's in your hands whether or not you do anything to halt the ageing process: nothing is for nothing. To reap the benefits you must first expend a little effort. Reading this book will not make you fit. Exercise works. But only if you work at it.

Of course you have to temper your judgement (and new-found enthusiasm) with a bit of mercy – i.e., common-sense. The fifty-five-year-old who aspires to take on his twenty-three-year-old junior at squash and beat him is asking for trouble, not to mention an elevated stress level and a possible heart attack. Try to keep things in perspective. You should aim to be the best you can be, not to be better than everybody else. Being fit at fifty is not a competition.

However, with a proper, balanced fitness regime which covers the three Ss of strength, stamina and suppleness, there is no earthly physiological reason why any moderately healthy fifty-year-old cannot find a new mid-term lease of life. This is because exercise makes the heart more efficient and the body stronger. It increases the range of motion, lowers stress levels, raises the spirits, helps you sleep more soundly, builds up the immune system and pumps oxygen into the extremities. All this improves skin, hair and overall body image. It can also act as preventative medicine against age-related diseases such as osteoporosis (thinning of the bones), angina and – provided body-weight exercise such as running is avoided – arthritis.

What exercise should not be is an end in itself. The elitist attitude of exercise for its own sake is not what *Fit to be 50* is all about. Exercise is a means to an end: that end is to live life to the full. Regular exercise allows you to overindulge now and again, to eat Christmas pudding, to have an occasional glass or two of wine of an evening. And though it needs to be built into the body-servicing routine (like cleaning your teeth) until it becomes a habit, it should not be a nasty habit like taking medicine. Believe it or not, exercise can be fun. It depends on choosing a discipline you enjoy, being motivated and sticking to it.

It also means taking no notice of those who say 'why bother?', 'it doesn't work', 'you look fine as you are'. It's not how you look, it's how you feel. And if you feel good you will look good. Just because some people give up doesn't mean you have to. Some people will not only never be fit at fifty they've probably never been fit in their lives. And they don't know what they're missing. They are the sort of people who always have an excuse, posing as a reason, why they shouldn't make an effort. Like that hoary old chestnut which says that if you take up exercise, when you give it up you will 'run to fat'. This is the purest nonsense. If you take up exercise and then quit, the worst thing that will happen is that you will go back to the state you were in before you started.

The problem is, where you were originally will feel fatter, unhealthier, more depressing than it did before. Because during the time you have been exercising, you will have come to realise perhaps for the first time since you were a child what it feels like to be truly alive.

Being fit is feeling young and it's never too late to start. That's why so many people don't give up once they've begun, not because they're afraid of going to seed – simply because regular exercise makes you feel on top of the world.

Here are some of the plusses of keeping fit at fifty. It will relieve tension and lift depression. So if you're menopausal, or if you're suffering the stress-load of a mid-life crisis at work, a work-out will make life easier to bear, not only for you, but for the poor unfortunates around who have to put up with you.

Activity boosts your metabolism, so you use up food more efficiently. As we get older the metabolic rate drops. This means we need less food to stay the same weight. If we go on eating as normal, little by little the weight will creep up – hence middle-age spread.

Exercise will keep you slim, trim, toned up and eating properly, which adds to the enjoyment of living and the feeling of living well. Working out not only makes you feel great now, it also acts as insurance for later on. It fortifies both the muscles and the skeleton underneath. It also keeps you flexible – movement is life, so keep moving. If you stop you'll stiffen up, your range of motion will decrease and this will, in turn, erode your independence. You owe it to yourself to take responsibility for your own body and keep yourself out of nursing homes for as long as possible, hopefully forever.

Being fit puts you in control of your own destiny. If your body is the servant rather than the master, then you are at liberty to change its shape and its capabilities, re-form it in the image that you would like, rather than put up with what you were given. And you *can* change your body. If aerobic exercise promotes overall fitness and reduces body fat, then resistance training (with or without weights) will improve your general shape. Strategic use of specific exercises will whittle your waist, tone up your thighs, slim down a heavy rear and/or build up your bust (by strengthening the pectoral muscles underneath). You can't alter your bone structure or add to your height, but cleverly distributed muscle will balance your silhouette, while streamlined thighs will give an illusion of longer legs.

Being fit allows you to live life to the full. It means you don't have to deny yourself those pleasures which make life worth living. All-round fitness is the greatest feeling there is. And thankfully more and more people are discovering this basic truth every day: you could be one of those people. Even if the closest you've ever been to getting fit is buying this book, you've made a start.

We are all the centre of our own universe. If your centre is supple and strong, then your particular universe will be the kind of quality place that it's a joy to inhabit. The benefits of being fit to be fifty are within your grasp! All you have to do is reach out – and turn over.

PART ONE
BODY MAINTENANCE

CHAPTER 1
GETTING ORGANISED

So what do you need to get started? Basically, just your body, your enthusiasm and an invisible piece of string (more of which later). You might also have a couple of bags of beans to hand and perhaps, but not necessarily, a child's skipping rope. Here is a list of the things you should have to get your *Fit to be 50* improvement plan underway.

1 **Space** Few of us have the luxury of a custom-built gym to which to retire to do the daily push-ups, but what you *will* need is space to move without damaging yourself or the priceless vase on the mantelpiece. Take a few minutes to shift the furniture out of the way before you get going. You'll need enough room to stretch your arms out at shoulder height, to stand on tip-toe and reach for the ceiling, and to lie down with your arms stretched above your head. If you have a garden and the weather is warm, you might like to work out outside. In this instance, though, unless you want to provide free entertainment for the entire neighbourhood, it's best to wear something modest and make sure you're not overlooked. Remember too that if you're doing aerobics, an unyielding surface is very hard on the joints, so it is better to work on the lawn rather than the patio.

2 **Time** Half an hour a day, six days a week. Try to fit this in when it's convenient so that you don't have any excuse not to do it. Write it in your diary as though it was a regular – and unbreakable – appointment: your appointment with you. Take the telephone off the hook. Give some consideration as to whether you're an owl or a lark. If you're a night person, then obviously you're not going to be at your best at 6.00 a.m., so work out in the evening. Similarly, if you're a lark, you'll be nodding off by 7.00 p.m. so get up half an hour early to get the most benefit. If you're out at work all day and don't have a gym where you can go for half an hour at lunchtime, then do your half-hour the minute you come in. Don't sit down: you'll never get up again.

3 **Music** They say that if you can remember the sixties you weren't there! Joking aside, our generation is lucky enough to have some wonderfully evocative music. Think of the selection: everything from The Beatles, through The Carpenters to The Beach Boys. So dig your old EPs out of the attic. Put them on the turntable and get started.

4 **Equipment** You need a duvet and a couple of cushions: the former to lie on when you are doing your post-exercise relaxation, the latter to protect vulnerable parts like your back or your knees while you are doing the floor exercises. Have a small towel handy, to wipe the sweat from your fevered brow.

5 **Shoes** Probably the most important item in an exercise buff's wardrobe, and the first thing you should invest in

should you decide to take up a sport seriously. There are specialist shoes for all sports, and it's wrong to think that a running shoe, for instance, will double up for an aerobics class. In a running shoe the maximum cushioning is on the heel; this is the part which hits the ground first when you run. In aerobic dance the ball of the foot makes contact first. So in a well-designed aerobic shoe the cushioning is located just forward of the instep. In both cases, correct shoes will support the foot and ankle, keep them stable on an uneven surface and cushion the shock of impact which otherwise travels right up through the ankle and knee joints to the hips and back. Working out on hard roads or unsprung floors in unsuitable shoes will leave you open to the onslaught of arthritis. Don't chance it. If you decide to swim or cycle instead on aerobic days, of course none of this will apply. On alternate days when you are doing body-conditioning work, you don't need shoes at all. Let your feet breathe for a change.

6 **Tracksuit** This is not so much an essential as a way of life. You can get an ordinary cotton tracksuit in an inspiringly bright colour (amazing how a canary yellow job can make you feel a hundred per cent better on a miserable March day) in any High Street chain store for a reasonable price.

Always wear a tracksuit to warm up. If you wear a T-shirt underneath you can strip the top off afterwards. Tracksuits are also handy for walking the dog, watering the garden or doing the weekly shop. And for leisure lounging they must be the most comfortable garment ever invented. If you don't have a tracksuit and don't want to buy one, then anything loose and comfortable will do. Avoid anything restricting, like wide belts or skintight jeans which will make it hard for you to breathe and limit your range of motion.

Those are what you *do* need.
These are what you *don't* need.

1 **Expensive Home Exercise Equipment** There must be more bullworkers and cross-country ski machines and hula hoops languishing under beds across the country than there are old socks. This is basically because working with a machine is boring. At the risk of alienating every exercise machine manufacturer in the business, I would like to go on record here and say that exercise bikes and rowing machines should be relegated to gymnasiums. There you can at least talk to your next-door neighbour while you are putting in your twenty minutes' worth. Twenty minutes' mindless pedalling can seem like three hours. Of course you can always wear a headset or watch TV to relieve the monotony, but this will distance you from your body rather than bringing you more in touch with it. And, since boredom is one of the biggest factors in abandoning an exercise regime, in my opinion, machines can do more harm than good when it comes to encouraging people to get up and go.

Some people feel that by making an investment in a piece of expensive equipment they will be committed to using it. Among my pupils I have invariably found the opposite to be the case. When they fall by the wayside they feel guilty every time they see the wretched machine. Boredom and guilt are two very negative emotions. They have no place in our *Fit to be 50* routine, or in our new lifestyle.

2 **Leotard and tights** You don't actually

need these for a home exercise routine. However, if it makes you feel better, why not? Gone are the days when work-out wear came in two colours, black or nothing, and some of the outfits on offer now are practically edible they are so delicious. So if you would like to join a weekly exercise class and/or feel that indulging in a figure-hugging bodysuit will focus you on your new body image, go ahead . You should avoid the current trend for things like bicycle shorts and keyhole cut-outs. These extreme fashions only look good on the very young. If you are spoiled for choice and don't know where to start, elasticised cotton is the best bet in materials. It's comfortable, doesn't wrinkle and absorbs sweat.

For those men among us, who I assume won't be wearing leotards, a word of warning: you shouldn't work out in shorts. Unless it is very hot, by exposing your bare legs you are leaving yourself open to cramp. If you have ever suffered from cramp then you'll know why I advise against tempting provi-dence. If you have never suffered from cramp you don't want to start now. For alternative lower body wear, try track-pants or pyjamas.

3 **Oils and Unguents** Again, these are non-essentials, but they can be very comforting for the first few weeks when you may find (especially if the most energetic thing you've done in the last twenty years is climb into the car) that parts of you are suffering from post-exercise stiffness. The Body Shop do some wonderful essential-oil-based rubs which you can massage into the back of your legs or wherever you need to loosen things up. Otherwise baby oil is perfectly acceptable. It is the massaging, rather than the oil, which does you good. If you're working out with your partner you can always massage each other. As we get older we tend to touch less, and take each other for granted more. Over the years this can lead to the point where it's difficult to know how to get started again: a gentle massage can be the perfect beginning.

CHAPTER 2

WARM-UP

Nothing banishes the blues or gets the circulation going like a good strong work-out. However, you *must* warm-up before you start. If you don't, you are leaving yourself open to the risk of serious injury, because cold muscles are tense muscles. Cold muscles are tight, and don't 'take the strain' and 'give' like long, lean, warm muscles do. Cold muscles *snap*. So don't skimp on your warm-up: it's important.

Before any kind of hard, deep muscle work it is vital to get that blood flowing and pump oxygen into the body, gently. Ease yourself in gradually, lubricating the joints and loosening up the main muscle groups, working right through from the top of the head to the tips of the toes until the entire body takes on a tingling glow. Then – and only then – is it safe to launch into the real hard work.

Incidentally, not only is it important to warm up initially, you need to stay warmed up. Several layers of light clothing are more efficient at doing this than a single heavy one. Air circulates between the layers, working on the 'wet-suit' principle: the temperature of the body warms the circulating air/water which in turn keeps the body warm. Natural fibres such as wool or cotton are better insulators than man-made fibres, and allow the body to sweat.

The rule of thumb for warming up is that you should perform the moves you aim to use in your work-out proper, but more slowly, with less intensity and using a smaller range of motion. Thus, even if your exercise routine consists merely of a leisurely turn round the links, you should do some upper body warm-ups such as arm circling and gentle trunk rotations before you leave the clubhouse. The classic twist and lift movement of a good golf swing, performed cold, has undoubtedly put many backs out.

Runners or walkers should correspondingly concentrate on the lower body, particularly the large muscle groups of the legs and buttocks. Jogging on the spot and side-to-side-pliés (performed with the back straight, the bottom tucked under and the knees kept over the feet for support) are good ways to ease the body into action.

Here are some gentle warm-up exercises which will prepare you for your *Fit to be 50* routine proper. You should do them every day, regardless of whether it is an aerobics or body conditioning day. That way you'll minimise the risk of injury and maximise the efficiency of your whole exercise routine.

Choose your own motivating music, but 'Here Comes the Sun' by The Beatles has the tempo for which you should be aiming: bright but not too fast. Also, although it's advisable to vary your music in general – to prevent your brain going onto automatic pilot – it's a good idea always to use the same music for your warm-up. As soon as you put it on and the first chord sounds, you'll be straight into your routine: reflex action. And, since getting started is the hardest part, every little helps.

So, music maestro please . . .

*B*IG BREATHS

The body can exist for months without food, days without water, but only minutes without air. So get some air into your lungs. Breathe deep and energise your body. Begin your routine (and your day) by taking four really deep breaths.

Standing tall, with feet hip-width apart, shoulders relaxed and arms hanging loosely by your sides, breathe in through the nose, simultaneously raising the arms up and out to the side, pressing the backs of the hands up and bringing the upper arms in towards the ears.

Now breathe out through the mouth, clearing all the stale air from the bottom of your lungs while pressing down with the palms of the hands and bringing the arms back to their original position.

Do this four times then shake the shoulders out and go on to the next exercise.

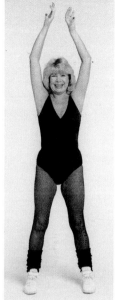

*R*EACH FOR THE SKY

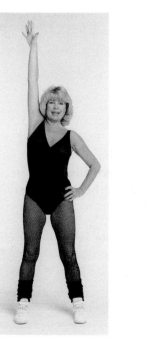

Keeping the knees soft and the tummy pulled in and up under the rib-cage, reach with alternate hands for the sky.

Do two sets of eight.

Really *stretch* up, spreading the fingers, aiming the tips up towards the ceiling. Keep the bottom tucked under so as not to arch the back and be careful not to twist the body.

SWINGTIME

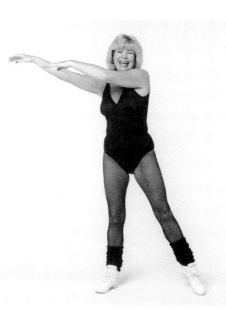

Swing both arms alternately from side to side while you step and touch your opposite foot on the ground.

Do eight on each side.

Be sure to keep the pelvis facing front and reach to the side so as not to twist the spine.

BOTTOM LINE

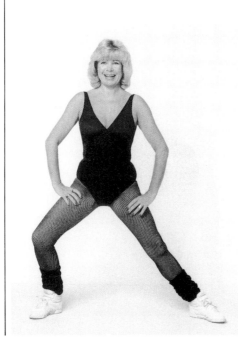

Begin with feet slightly wider than hip-width apart, knees soft, toes turned out at the diagonal.

Now, keeping the knees pushed back over the feet, the back straight and the bottom tucked under, lunge rhythmically from side to side.

Do eight on each side, taking care not to bring the knee any further than level with the foot each time.

Shake out the legs and continue.

SPINE STRETCHERS

Standing with knees and feet hip-width apart, feet parallel, bend the knees and tuck the bottom under. Press tail bone down towards the floor in small, pulsing movements for a count of eight.

Ease the right shoulder gently down towards the right knee. Make small pulsing movements for a count of eight. Release and repeat on the other side.

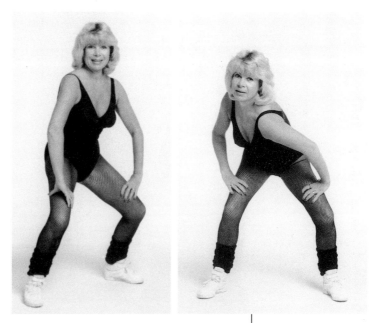

TOE TAPS

Keeping the knees bent and the heels on the ground, raise the toes of the right foot up towards the right knee. Tap and raise the toes eight times. You should feel it in your shin and calves. Repeat the movement eight times with the left foot.

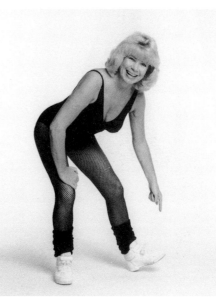

SHOULDER ROLLS

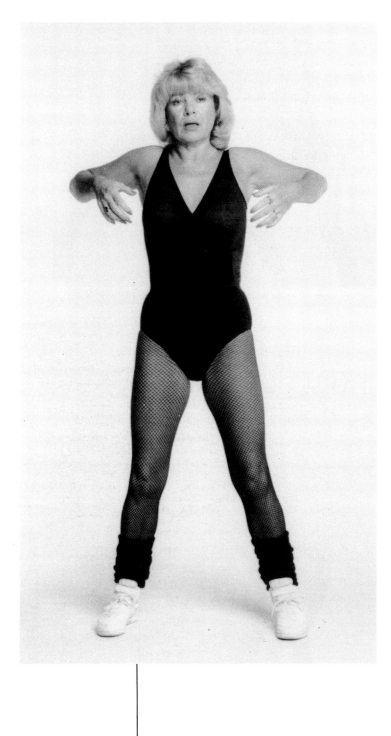

Slowly rotate the shoulders up and back in a big circle. First ease them up towards the ears, then try to press the shoulder-blades together at the back, and finally bring them down, forward and up and to their original position.

Complete four circles going backwards, then reverse the movement and do four coming forwards.

SCOOPS

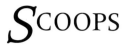

First, do a 'three-point pull': pull the points of your shoulders down to the floor, while easing the crown of your head up towards the ceiling. You should feel a lengthening sensation in your neck.

Allow the chin to drop forward to the point that, when you look at the floor, your eyes connect with a spot about a foot forward from your toes.

Scoop your head to the right until the point of the chin is over the point of the right shoulder. Now tilt the chin up, aiming it at the angle where the ceiling meets the wall. *Don't drop the head back.* If you're doing it right, you'll feel a 'pull' in the neck under the chin.

Hold for a count of eight, breathing regularly and evenly throughout, then reverse the movement, bringing the chin over the point of the right shoulder and tipping up as before.

Make two more of these sweeping movements across the chest, finishing with the head in the centre. Raise the head slowly and relax.

Finish your warm-up by walking briskly round the room three or four times before you launch into the routine proper.

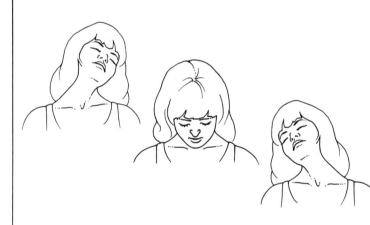

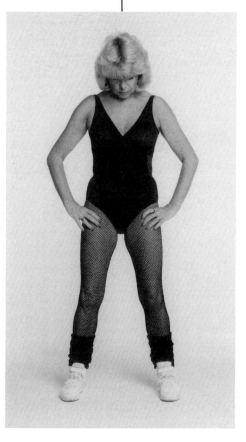

CHAPTER 3
AEROBICS

You *must* do twenty minutes' worth of aerobics every other day, but you don't necessarily have to do the exercises that follow. There are more ways than one to get your aerobic exercise.

Running is an aerobic exercise; so are cycling, swimming, and good, old-fashioned walking, which none of us do enough of these days. If you're a time-and-motion devotee, and looking for ways to build a routine into your lifestyle, you could easily cover your aerobic days by cycling to work or walking to the shops instead of taking the car. If you normally go by bus, then think of walking there and coming back the usual way.

If your job is close to a swimming pool, then you might like to do your twenty minutes (warm up in the changing room) first thing in the morning or straight after work. Otherwise try swimming in your lunch hour once in a while. Incidentally, never work out on a full stomach, or under the influence of alcohol or drugs. The latter is dangerous since you won't be in control and could risk injury. The former is inadvisable as your system will have gone into 'food-digesting mode'; if you try to exercise you will feel not only uncomfortably full, but possibly quite sick. You should leave a good two hours between eating and exercising.

Swimming is one activity which is suitable for anyone of any age, as the water cushions the body weight. If you have problems with your knees or ankles it is a very safe way of using the muscles without putting any strain on the joints. The resistance of the water makes swimming an extremely effective discipline, and you don't even need to be one of those enviable water babies capable of executing a perfect Australian crawl to get results. The breast-stroke is just as effective, and has the added advantage of improving the bustline, or chest, by strengthening the pectoral muscles which support it.

If you are one of those people who gets bored easily, you can mix and match your routines – cycling in the springtime, perhaps, and swimming in the summer. You could walk in the autumn when the leaves are beginning to fall, and do your exercises inside during the cold winter months. Otherwise you could swop disciplines once a month, or do something different on each aerobic day. Remember, though, that sports such as tennis and squash are *not* aerobic. They may be energetic, but the energy is expended in fits and starts. To maintain aerobic status you must first raise the heart rate, and then keep it raised for a minimum of twenty minutes.

If you opt for an exercise class at a local facility, keep in mind that Low Impact Aerobics (LIA) is much kinder to joints and pelvic floors than High Impact Aerobics (HIA). It is also much more effective for burning body fat. Current research has shown that aerobic activity carried out at lower intensity for a longer period of time is more effective at shifting unwanted flab than higher intensity exercise carried out for a shorter period. In other words, if you're trying to reduce body fat it's better to go for a forty-minute walk than a twenty-minute run.

But why do aerobics at all? Well, basically because aerobic (which literally means 'with air') fitness improves life expectancy. The heart, which is a muscle, is made more efficient by the aerobic process; since heart disease is the big twentieth-century killer, it makes sense to take out a little aerobic insurance. The stroke volume (the amount of blood pumped through the system with each heartbeat) increases with what is known as 'the training effect'. Because of this, the stroke rate (the number of times the heart pumps per minute) decreases. A really healthy heart can pump up to twenty times less per minute than an unhealthy one. It stands to reason that the less strain you put on the heart the longer it – and ultimately you – will last. As we become aerobically fit, a greater amount of oxygen is taken in and utilised with each breath. This not only improves our overall health, it also has a positive cosmetic effect.

Doing aerobic exercise improves the circulation and gives the skin a healthy glow, it makes the eyes sparkle and the hair shine. Well-being becomes something that comes from within, so that we need no longer rely on outside influences, like the weather or other people's attitudes, to make us feel good. If we look great, we feel great; since being fit will *make* you feel great, you will build up your self-confidence and have the energy and drive to tackle things (and succeed!) that you would never have attempted during your lethargic old pre-exercise days.

How do you know whether or not you're doing enough? To achieve the 'training effect' you need to work out regularly. So far as the level of activity is concerned, you should be able to carry on a conversation while you are working out. You should be pleasantly out of breath, but not breathless.

If you are puce in the face and feel as though you aren't going to make it through the next minute, you are clearly doing too much too soon. Be sensible, and slow down. If you feel dizzy, faint or sick, or have any pains in your chest you should, of course, stop straight away. When you feel better you should go straight to the telephone and make an appointment with your doctor for a check-up. That said, everyone should get out of breath at least once a day. If you can't climb a couple of flights of stairs or run to catch the bus without feeling as though your last hour has come, you are *seriously* out of condition. The sooner you start an aerobic routine the better.

How about *now*?

STAIR STEPPING

Stand at the bottom of the stairs, knees and feet together, arms hanging loose. Step up on the first tread – right foot followed by left. Now step down again.

Continue this brisk 'stepping' movement for two minutes changing the lead foot after the first minute.

Increase stamina by adding one minute per week to your daily stepping time up to a maximum of five minutes.

Since this is essentially a repetitive exercise, keep motivation high by playing music with a good strong beat.

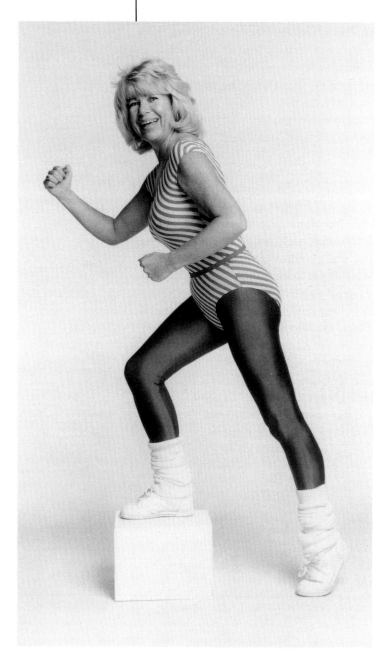

*P*OINT AND PRESS

Step from side to side, pointing the toes
and stretching the leg. At the same time,
interlock the fingers and push the flat of
the hands down towards the floor. Each
time you press, imagine you are trying to
squeeze an extra sweater into a drawer
which is already too full.

Keep pointing and pressing for four
counts of eight.

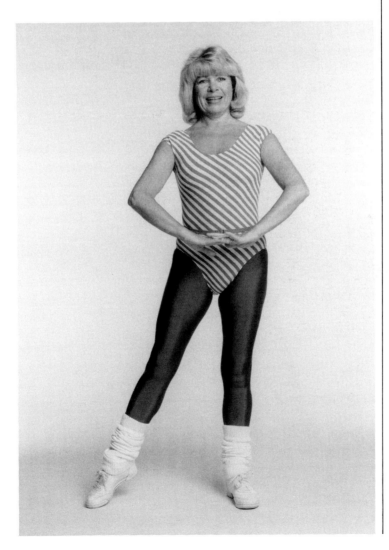

HEEL AND HAUL

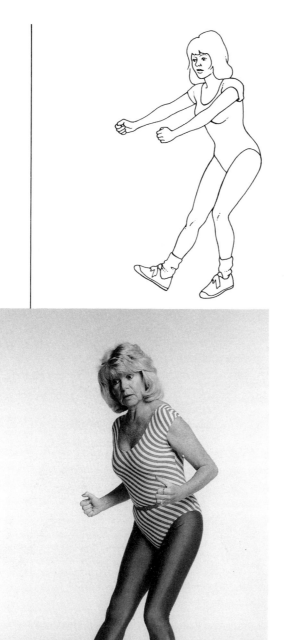

Step forward with alternate feet, pressing the heel down into the ground each time.

Simultaneously, reach forward with both hands as though grasping something, and then haul them back hard, pressing the shoulder blades together at the back with each pull.

Keep the arms close to the sides and try not to hunch the shoulders.

Do four sets of eight.

PRESS BACKS

Reach feet back, one at a time, touching toes to the floor. Try not to bend the knee, and be careful not to arch the lower back. Keep the stomach pulled in and up to support and stabilise the trunk.

Now raise the arms to shoulder height and press them back each time you stretch the leg. If you are doing it right you will feel a pull across the front of the chest, level with the armpit. Make the movements large but controlled. Don't fling your arms about wildly.

Do four more sets of eight.

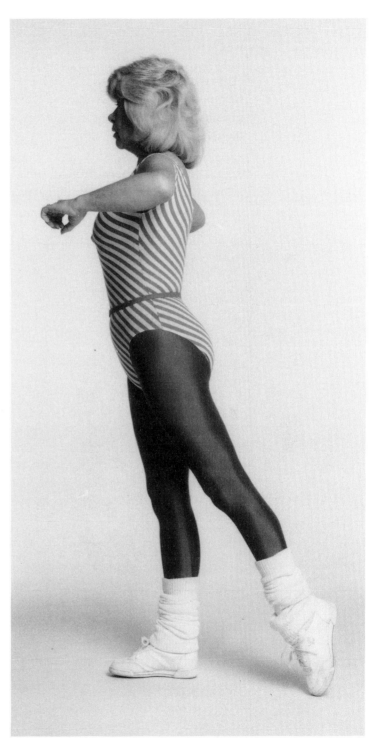

PULL-DOWNS

Standing tall with feet hip-width apart, reach up towards the ceiling with fingers spread.

Now pull the elbows down sharply while simultaneously raising one knee towards the chest.

Repeat this movement twelve times, using alternate legs and breathing normally throughout.

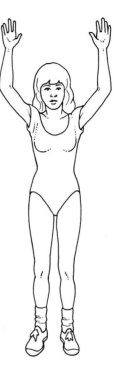

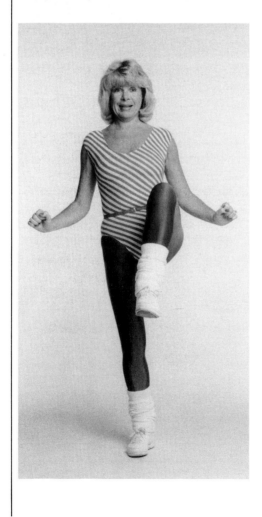

COCKADOODLE ROCKS

Keeping feet parallel, but with one foot about eighteen inches ahead of the other, rock backwards and forwards rocking horse fashion. At the same time flap your arms up and down like wings.

Do two sets of eight with your right foot forward then change legs and do two more sets.

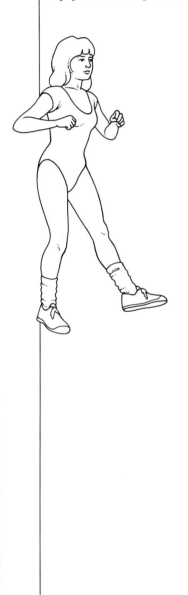

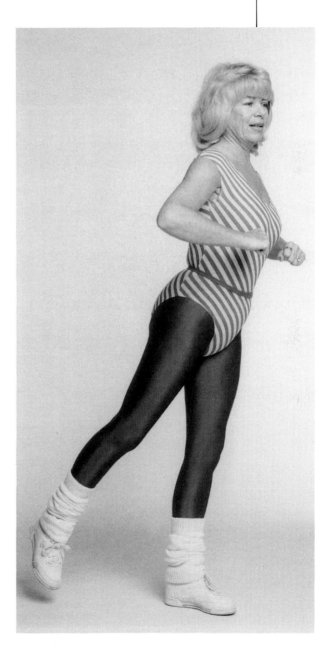

SKIP

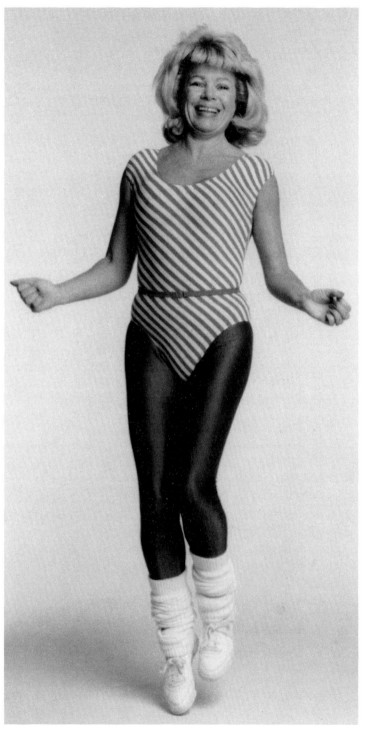

Pick up the skipping rope I mentioned at the beginning of chapter one and get cracking. Twenty times forward, twenty times back, gradually working up to a hundred each way as your stamina improves. If you don't have a skipping rope, simply hold your upper arms in close to your body and pretend.

Keep the feet low and move from foot to foot rather than jumping and landing on both feet at the same time. It's easier on the joints. If you have problems with your pelvic floor, you may want to leave this one out.

SIMON SAYS

Jogging on the spot, place the hands on the shoulders and raise them up and down towards the ceiling for two sets of eight. Keep jogging and, without allowing the arms to drop below shoulder height, stretch them forwards and back for two sets of eight.

Open the arms in and out to the side for two sets of eight, making sure that only the lower arms move. Hold the upper arms steady and parallel to the floor. Breathe regularly and evenly throughout this sequence.

When you have finished, shake the shoulders out to relieve any tension, and then do the whole thing over again.

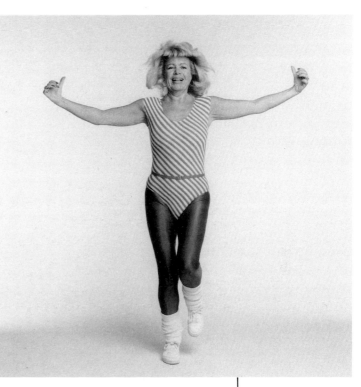

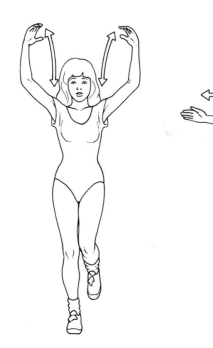

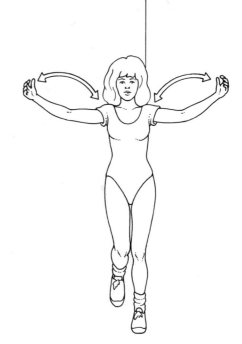

33

HAND JIVE

Take two steps to the right, followed by two steps to the left (bringing you back to where you started). Keep moving like this, in rhythm with the music, and do the hand jive.

Keep your upper arms close to your body, palms facing the floor and fingers spread wide. Do as many as you like, a whole chorus if you're having fun.

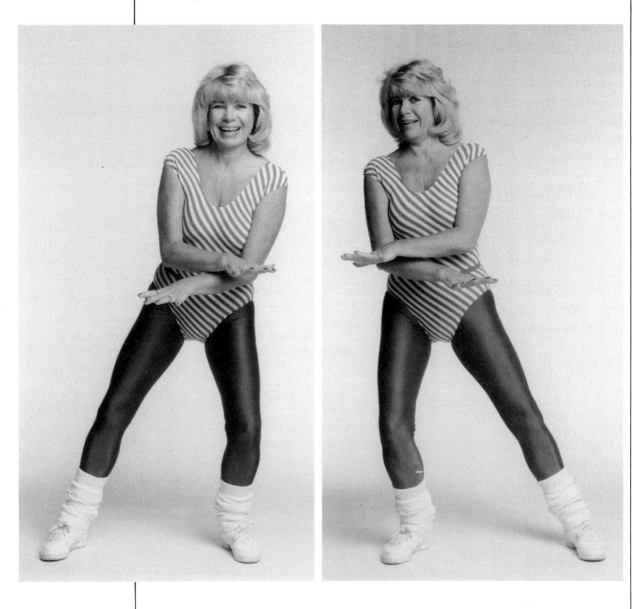

POWER WALKING

March briskly round the room, the house, the garden, driving the knees up towards the chest and swinging the arms vigorously. Hold the hands in loose fists, palms turned in towards the face and 'pump' them up towards the ceiling. Don't walk on the toes, rather bring the whole of the foot down with each stride. Continue 'power walking' for three to four minutes, breathing deeply for maximum oxygen intake. (Note: because there is no momentum involved – as there would be if you were running – and you are having to raise each leg using only your muscle power, you will find that this exercise is much harder than it looks. A bit like wading through glue.)

At the end of your routine, walk around the room, three or four times, swinging your arms in big circles and bringing your speed down gradually. Never stop dead or the blood may pool in your feet and make you feel light-headed. When your breathing has returned to normal go on to the stretch section (see Chapter 5).

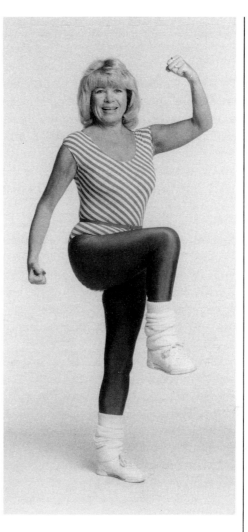

CHAPTER 4
BODY CONDITIONING

Body conditioning won't help you lose weight. What it *will* do is make you look as though you've lost weight by tightening up the floppy bits (under-arm and inner thigh), neatening the waist and generally lending definition to the body line. An added advantage is that you can tailor your routine to your own individual needs. If you're the classic English pear-shape, for example, then exercises for the lower body will neaten your seat and streamline your thighs. Corresponding upper body work will strengthen the shoulders and chest, giving the whole torso a more balanced aspect.

The exercises which follow are designed to condition the entire body. You should do them on alternate days.

If you have a particular problem, such as floppy inside thighs or a spare tyre, then you can do twice as many of the relevant exercise than is recommended for general body toning.

For upper body work you can add the extra resistance of a 1lb bag of beans, held in each hand, if you like. To strengthen a muscle you must first overload it, and this extra weight will make your muscles work harder and give you faster results. I recommend that you don't use cans since, if you drop one on your foot from shoulder height, it can give you a very sore toe. If you are extremely unfit, be gentle on yourself; don't add weights until you've been doing the programme regularly for at least a couple of months. The old adage of 'no pain, no gain' is very, very dangerous. Little and often is the rule with any exercise. If you do too much too soon you will get stiff and sore and give up, which is the last thing any of us wants.

You will see that I've recommended a certain number of sets (a set is eight repetitions) for each exercise. This is meant to be used as a guideline only. If you can't manage the whole thing at first, don't despair: just do your best. As you get stronger you'll be able to add more repetitions until, before you know it, you'll be sailing through it all. Similarly, if you are in reasonably good condition and don't feel challenged by the routine, then add an extra few repetitions wherever and whenever you like.

Whatever exercise you are doing, never work through pain, specifically pain in the neck or the lower back. Pain is the body's way of telling you to stop. These exercises are designed to be as safe as current physiological research can make them, so if you feel pain you are either doing them wrong or you are doing too much too soon. Listen to your body; it's the only one you've got.

Incidentally, since it's almost impossible to perform an exercise and read the instructions at the same time (unless you're a professional contortionist, in which case you hardly need my help!) it might be an idea to enlist the aid of someone to read the instructions aloud to you the first time you attempt the exercises. It also helps if you work in front of a full-length mirror for a week or so, just to make sure you're in the correct positions. With strength exercises you need to be specific in your placing of the body, otherwise you may not be reaching the right muscles and it would be a shame if you didn't get maximum value for your efforts.

Apart from the aesthetic aspects, body conditioning – or resistance training as it's sometimes called – also makes your muscles stronger. This in turn guards against joint injury. For instance, the recommended way to lift a heavy weight is to hug it close to the body and stand up straight using the thigh muscles as a pushing off point. If these quadriceps muscles, which run down the front of the thigh, aren't strong enough (and in women especially they are notoriously weak), this simply isn't possible. The individual bends to lift the weight and the back takes the strain. The result is a pulled muscle or, in extreme cases, a damaged disc. Strong stomach muscles, girdling the torso like a corset, also pro-tect the back. For this reason, no matter how much of a rush you're in, you should try to fit some stomach exercises into each and every session.

Happy exercising!

TUMS

The trouble with tums is that they get less natural exercise than any other part of the body. We walk around on our legs and pick up things with our arms so we're bound to have some muscles in those particular areas. But the main thing we do with the stomach is put food inside it.

The other trouble with tums is that one exercise alone won't do the necessary tightening and toning. There are several distinct sets of tummy muscles and it stands to reason that to strengthen them all you'll need several distinct sets of exercises.

CURL-UPS

Curl-ups are great for the spare tyre, and have replaced the old fashioned 'sit-up' which is unsafe for the back and, performed with the feet hooked under a chair, can cause the muscles to bulge and produce a pot belly.

Lie flat on your back with arms loosely by your sides. Knees up to the ceiling, feet flat on the floor and hip-width apart. Imagine someone is going to punch you in the solar plexus. Your muscles should tense and tighten in anticipation of the blow. Keep them like that. Don't hold your breath.

Now raise your hands towards the points of your knees. Keeping the tummy tight and the lower back pressed firmly into the floor, curl your head and shoulders up for a slow count of four, *simultaneously sliding your hands up your thighs*. Only come as high as is comfortable. You should feel no tension in the neck or upper back. Make the stomach do the work for you.

Hold at your highest point for a count of four. Then lower for a count of four. Breathe *out* as you come up, *in* as you relax.

Do as many curl-ups as is comfortable. Four is usually a safe number to begin with. As your stomach gets stronger you can increase the number by a couple every week until you're doing twenty.

SPINAL CURLS

Lie flat on your back; knees tucked in towards your chest, hands tucked under your behind. Now curl the knees in towards the chest in a series of small curls, bringing the lower back off the floor each time. Keep the tummy tight and flat.

Do eight to ten (they are *very* hard work), working up to twenty over a period of weeks.

Stretch out like a starfish to relax.

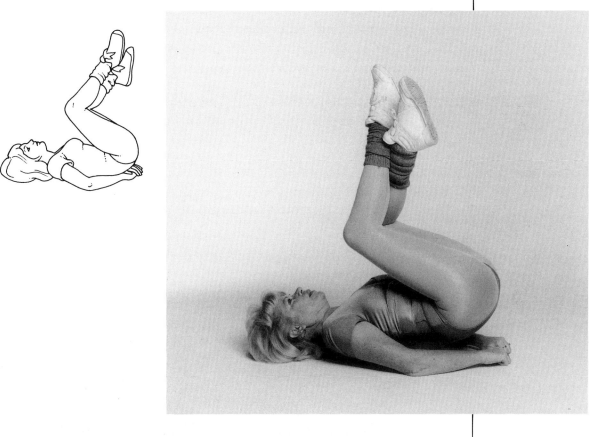

CROSS-OVERS

1. Lie flat on your back; knees tucked in on your chest; feet crossed at the ankles. Clasp your hands behind your head, winging your elbows out to the side.

2. Now raise your head and shoulders about an inch off the floor. Bring your hands round beside your ears (to avoid the temptation of pulling the head up with the hands as you raise the upper body). This is your resting position.

3. Pull the top half of your body up and round, aiming your left elbow towards your right knee.

Relax back to your resting position. Now aim the right elbow to the left knee. Repeat cross-overs for three counts of eight, twenty-four altogether. Only come as high as is comfortable. The 'twist' is more important than the 'lift'. Don't fret if you don't get near your knees at first. That will come with time and perseverance.

4. When you've finished, allow the head and shoulders to relax back onto the floor. Uncross your ankles and bring your feet down flat onto the floor. Now stretch your arms out in a T-shape and gently drop your knees first to one side, then to the other, to release any tension in the lower back.

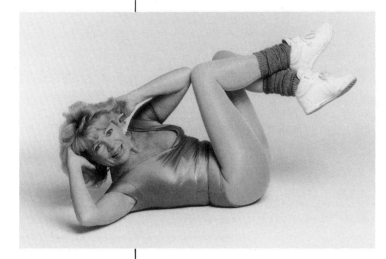

WOBBLY BITS

1. Lie supine with knees pointing towards the ceiling, feet flat on the floor, knees and feet hip-width apart. Press the back of the waist down, squeeze the bottom tight and tilt the pelvis up.

2. Stretch the arms out in a T-shape at shoulder height. Raise the arms an inch off the floor, palms facing the ceiling, elbows slightly bent, fingers curled in lightly.

3. Bring the hands in to meet each other at eye level, then out again. Do this eight times, concentrating on the inside of the upper arm.

4. Now, holding the arms *just* off the floor, make tiny little pushes up towards the ceiling for three sets of eight.

(If you want to make this exercise doubly effective you can add a pound bag of dried beans or lentils to each hand.)

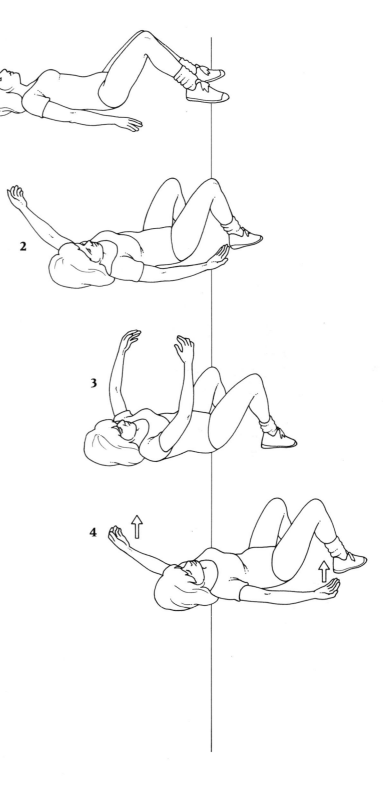

*B*OOBS

Staying in the same position, bringing your hands up towards the ceiling with the palms facing your feet and make big walks with the arms for a count of eight, taking care not to touch the floor either by your side or above your head.

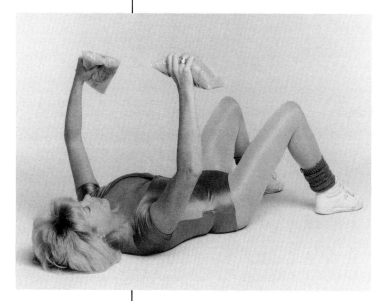

Then stretch *both* arms above the head, with elbows slightly bent, and interlock your thumbs. Now, keeping the backs of the hands as close to the floor as possible without actually touching it, push the arms upwards in small pulsing movements for three sets of eight.

Bring the arms down by your sides, shake the shoulders out and relax.

Note: don't hold your breath – especially if you are weighted – as this will push your blood pressure up. Instead, breathe in small puffs in time with each lift. If this is too confusing at first just breathe regularly and evenly, or count out loud, or sing along with the music.

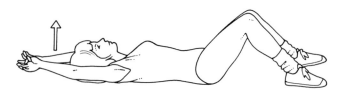

UNDER ARMS

Grab your bag of beans in each hand and, using a cushion to protect the kneecap, kneel on one knee. Make sure the thigh of the other leg is parallel to the floor with that knee placed directly over the foot for support. Lay the upper body across the thigh, keeping the neck in line with the back, upper arms tucked in by the sides, lower arms curled forward.

Unhinging them at the elbow, lift the lower arms up and back until the arm is almost fully extended. Now bend them back to their original position. Repeat for two sets of eight, increasing to four sets as you become stronger.

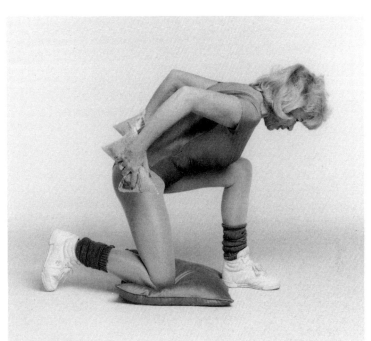

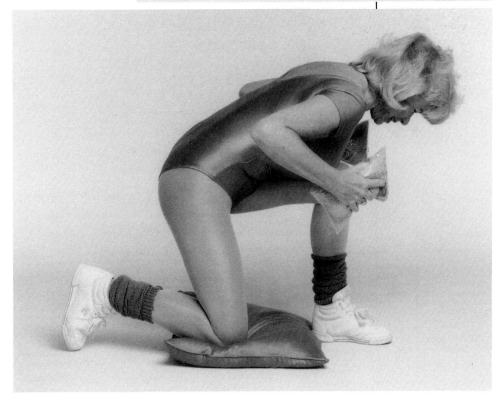

REAR VIEW

Begin on all fours, back straight, stomach pulled in tight. Raise one leg so that it is parallel to the floor. There should be one long continuous line from the base of the skull to the back of the heel.

Squeezing the bottom tight, drop the flexed foot downwards, stopping just before the toes reach the floor, then lift the leg back up to its original position. Raise and lower for two sets of eight. Change legs and repeat.

From the starting position you might find it more comfortable to come down onto the lower arms. Then raise one leg parallel to the floor and continue the exercise as above.

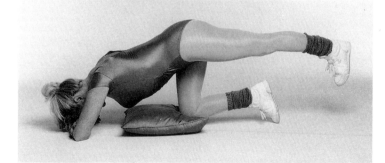

BOTTOMS UP

Start in the same position as for the previous exercise, the body weight distributed evenly. Now come down onto the lower arms to minimise any arch in the back. Relax neck and shoulders but keep tummy taut.

Raise the right leg until the thigh is parallel to the floor. Bend the knee keeping the flat of the foot facing the ceiling. Squeezing the bottom tight, push the back of thigh and flat of foot upwards towards the ceiling for three counts of eight. Rest and repeat with other leg.

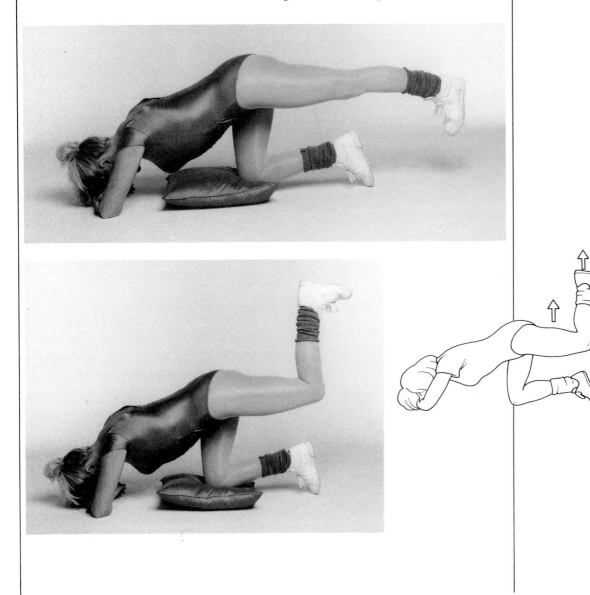

FRONT OF LEGS

1. Sit up straight, hands on the floor for support, knees and feet hip-width apart. Knees and flexed toes should be pointing up towards the ceiling.

2. Now press the backs of the knees down into the carpet and attempt to raise the heels off the floor. *Don't* lean back. Keep *both* heels off the floor throughout the exercise.

3. Lift the right leg a couple of inches and bend and stretch it for two counts of eight. Now straighten it and push it up towards the ceiling (one inch, no more) for two sets of eight.

4. Finally circle the entire leg in for eight, then out for eight. Lower leg. Repeat with left leg. Shake legs out. Relax.

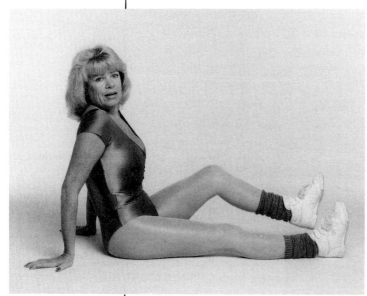

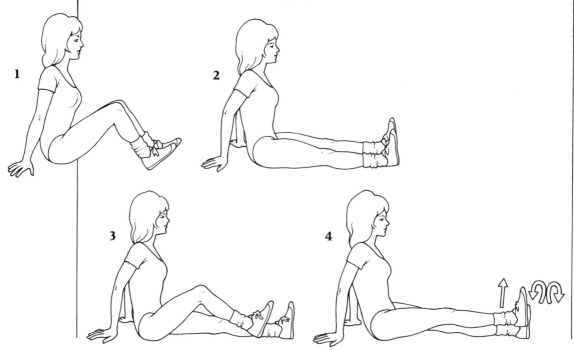

Note: this is pure muscle work: the harder it is the more you need it. This is because you are using the weight of your own legs to work the quadriceps muscles down the fronts of the thighs and the hip flexors on the sides.

Watch your form. Don't hold your breath, grit your teeth, hunch your shoulders or take your body weight on your hands. Make your legs do the work. It is better to do two of these right than fifty wrong.

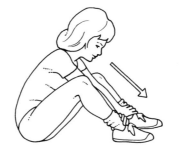

Stretch 1: sit up straight, knees up to the ceiling, feet flat on the floor. Knees and feet should be a hip-width apart. Slide the arms down the inside of the thighs, then wrap the hands round the ankles. Using the insteps for leverage, press the breastbone down towards the floor between the legs.

Stretch 2: roll over onto your right side, resting the body weight on the lower arm. Grasp the left ankle with the left hand and bring the heel in towards the buttocks. Don't pull in too hard, especially if you have knee problems. Instead press the foot *out* against the restraining hand. Now tilt your pelvis under and forward and you should feel a strong stretch down the front of the thigh. Hold for ten, change legs and repeat on the other side. Note: don't hold your breath.

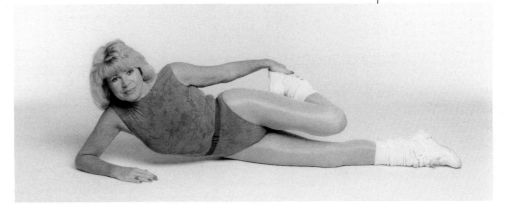

47

WAIST AWAY

Lie on your right side, upper body resting on the lower arm, legs parallel, feet crossed at the ankle. Press down with the left hand and raise the upper body off the floor so that there is a straight line from the ankle to the armpit.

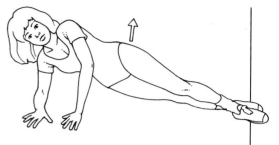

Imagine that an invisible piece of string (You wondered when we were getting to that, didn't you?) is attached to your hip bone and is pulling you up and down beneath the ceiling like a marionette. Don't tilt the body forward. If you're doing it right you should feel it in the underside of your waist.

Raise and lower the body for two sets of eight. Turn over and repeat.

Now roll over onto your back and stretch your arms along the floor above your head. Relaxing the left side of the body, stretch the fingers of the right hand and the toes of the right foot vigorously in opposite directions. Feel the stretch in the waist. Hold for a count of eight, breathing regularly and evenly. Relax the right side and repeat on the left.

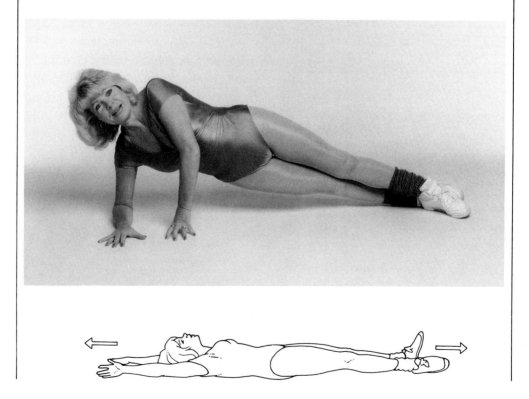

BACKS OF LEGS

Keeping the right foot flat, stretch the right leg out until there is only a gap of about twelve inches between the back of the knee and the floor. Place the left foot on the right thigh. Raise the bottom one inch off the floor.

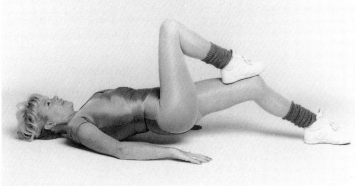

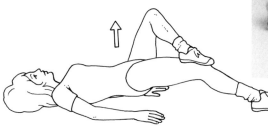

Lower and raise like this for two sets of eight.

Change sides and repeat.

Note: This is quite hard work. If you are doing it right you should feel it in the hamstring, which runs roughly from the behind to the back of the knee.

At this point it's a good idea to do a stretch.

Ease the right knee in towards the chest, being careful not to pull the bottom off the floor.

Hold for a count of eight, breathing regularly and evenly.

Now stretch the leg out and, holding on behind the knee and winging the elbows out to the side, press down with the hands and up with the leg at the same time. Hold for eight. Keep breathing! Don't tense the neck or shoulders and don't raise the head off the floor.

Relax and repeat both stretches with the other leg.

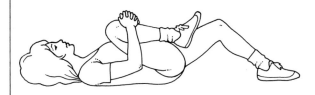

*I*NSIDE THIGH

Lie on your side, propped up on the elbow, legs stretched out. Raise the top leg up and over the lower one. Stretch the bottom leg out, flexing the toes. Raise this leg about an inch off the floor. This is your resting position.

With your ankle facing the ceiling raise the leg six inches then lower to the resting position again.

Repeat this action for two counts of eight, increasing to four counts as the muscles become stronger. Do the other leg, then shake out any tension and relax.

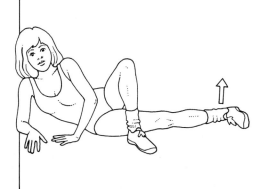

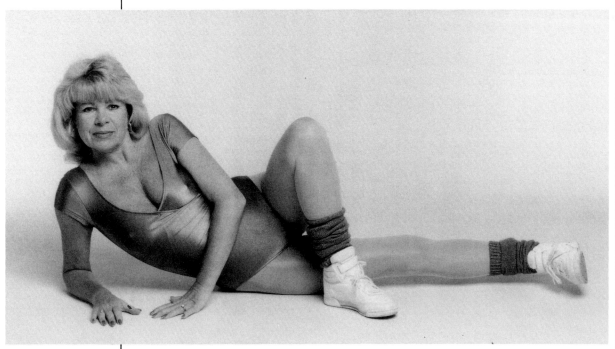

OUTSIDE THIGH

1. Lie on your side, legs parallel, toes flexed, head supported loosely in the hand. Bend the bottom leg at a right-angle to hold the back steady. Make sure to keep the upper leg stretched out with the ankle bone facing the ceiling.

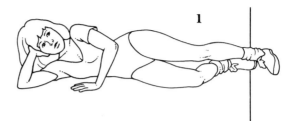

2. Now raise the upper leg an inch above the lower. From this position lift and drop the leg an inch each way for a count of sixteen.

Point the toes. Lift and lower for two more sets of eight.

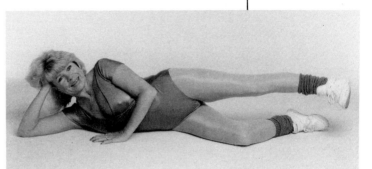

3. Finally do two sets of tiny bend stretches, pushing the flat of the foot away firmly with each stretch.

Shake the legs out to relieve any tension. Turn over and do the other side.

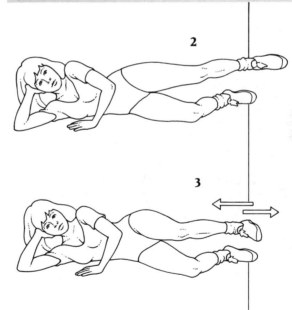

MINI PRESS-UPS

Rest on hands and knees with a cushion under the knees for support. Your hands should be under the points of the shoulders, knees together, feet crossed at the ankles and elbows slightly bent. Keep the lower legs (from knee to ankle) on the floor to avoid any pressure on the kneecap.

Tucking the pelvis forward so that there is a straight line from the shoulder to the back of the knee, bend the elbows and lower the upper body towards the floor. Now push up again.

Raise and lower ten times, breathing in as you come down, out as you come up.

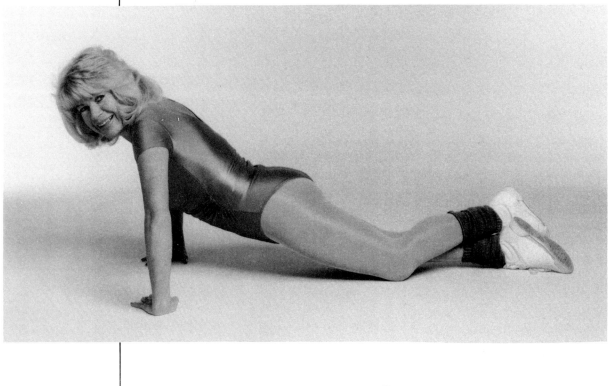

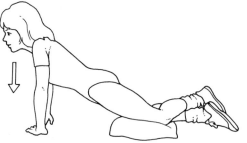

CHAPTER 5
STAY LOOSE

Supple equals young; stiff equals old. These are two excellent reasons to make sure your body is well stretched out. Some senior citizens have lost so much flexibility that they are incapable of tying their shoelaces or putting on their coats without assistance. In losing mobility, they have lost a much more precious commodity: independence.

Staying loose is especially important if you are a sportsperson. Aerobics will improve your cardiovascular system (heart and lungs), calisthenics will make your muscles strong, but unless you stretch those muscles out, they will snap rather than give the first time they are put under strain.

Men are generally much less flexible than women, which is hormonal. Women in childbirth obviously need to be reasonably loose (especially in the inner thigh and pelvic area) successfully to deliver a baby. Men, on the other hand, are usually stronger than women because they are able to build up more muscle – again because of hormones.

The tightest, stiffest parts of the body tend to be the neck and shoulders, upper and lower back, inner thighs and (if you are habitually in high heels) backs of legs.

The following are a few simple stretches aimed at increasing the flexibility of all these areas safely and effectively. As with the warm-up, you should do them every day, irrespective of whether you've been doing aerobics or body-conditioning.

A good stretch at the end of an exercise session minimises post exercise stiffness (PES), a little of which you will have to expect, especially if you are what the Americans call 'a couch potato'.

A word of advice before you begin. Try not to 'bounce' into a stretch. This is called a ballistic movement, and it is pointless. If you bounce you are simply 'pinging' your muscles in and out like an elastic band, not actually stretching them at all. To be effective a stretch needs to be *held* at the point of maximum resistance and the end of your normal range of motion; this should be done long enough for the muscles to lengthen, but never long enough so that it becomes painful.

The positions illustrated are the ones you should aim for. If you don't get anywhere near them to begin with, don't give up in disgust. Above all, don't strain or hold your breath, unless you want to push up your blood pressure. Repetition is the secret of effective stretching. The more you practise, the suppler you'll become. Never force yourself into an attitude that is uncomfortable. If you do, you'll do more harm than good.

Everyone is built differently: some people are lucky enough to be just naturally supple; most aren't. But over a period of time you will gradually increase your flexibility. It takes three months on average to stretch a body out. Have faith. Performed little and often, these exercises will supple you up.

TENSION RELEASE

If your work has you slaving over a hot stove (or word-processor), doing anything, in fact, which involves holding the shoulders in one position for any length of time, lactic acid can build up in the muscles in the back of the neck, causing stiffness which may well escalate into a tension headache. Since prevention is better than cure, use this little 'coping strategy' to nip the problem in the bud.

Stand up and clasp your hands together behind the back.

Do a 'three-point pull': that invisible piece of string is now attached to the crown of the head, pulling you upwards towards the ceiling. At the same time press the points of your shoulders down towards the floor. Feel the lengthening sensation in your neck.

Keeping your hands clasped, draw your shoulder-blades together and ease your upper arms towards each other across your back. Hold for a count of eight. Release and repeat.

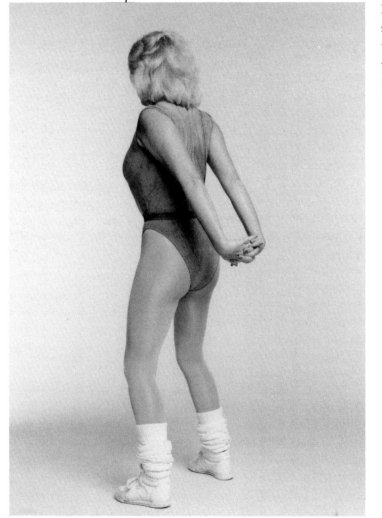

UPPER BACK STRETCH

Interlock the fingers in front of the body and, pressing the palms away from you, curve the back and bend the knees, invisible piece of string now attached to the back of your waist and pulling you towards the wall. Keep the tummy in tight and try not to hunch the shoulders.

Hold the stretch for a count of eight. Relax and repeat.

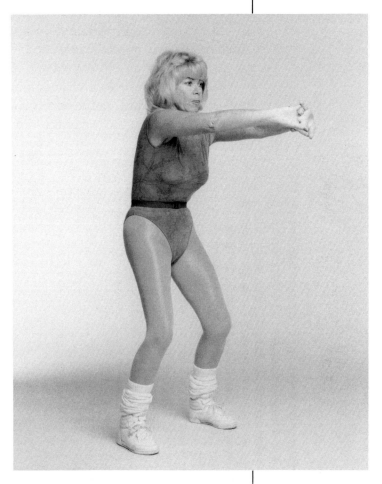

LOWER BACK

This stretch will iron out the kinks in the spine, and lengthen the erector spinae muscles and hip flexors. When these muscles are too tight, they can cause lower back curvature and a corresponding bulging belly.

Lie supine, knees up to the ceiling, feet flat on the floor, with neck and shoulders relaxed.

Pick up the right leg, slide the hands under the knee and hug the thigh down towards the chest. Try not to tense the shoulders or arch the neck. Hold for a count of eight. Relax. Pick up the left leg and repeat.

Finally bring both legs into the chest, hug them down and hold for two counts of eight. Replace feet in original position and move on to the next exercise.

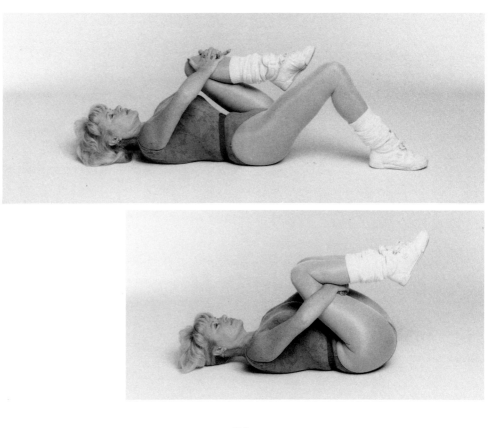

HIP FLEXORS AND HAMSTRINGS

Bring the right leg into your chest as you did in the last exercise, hugging the thigh as close to the body as you can without pulling your bottom off the floor.

Now unhinge the leg, aiming the shin towards the face. The thigh will move slightly further away from the chest. Don't worry about that.

Keeping the leg as straight as you can, pull the knee towards the nose while simultaneously pressing the leg up against the resistance of your hands. Don't hold your breath. If you're doing it right, the leg shouldn't move.

Hold for a count of eight. Release and repeat with the other leg.

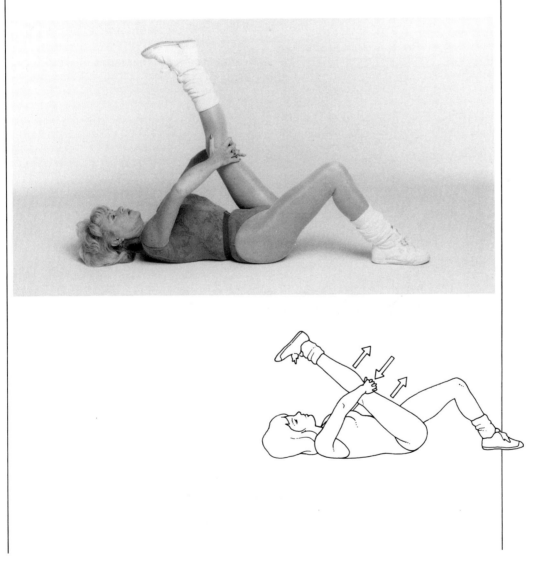

INNER THIGH AND CHEST RELAXER

Bring the knees and feet together. Knees up to the ceiling, feet flat on the floor.

Stretch the arms above your head allowing the backs of the hands to relax back into the floor. Feel the upper body opening out. Get rid of the tension by telling your arms to sink back into the floor.

Now allow the knees to drop open to the sides. Just as far as is comfortable. Feel the lower body opening out.

The whole body should now feel like a book which has dropped open at its centre page. Lie there and unwind for a slow count of eight.

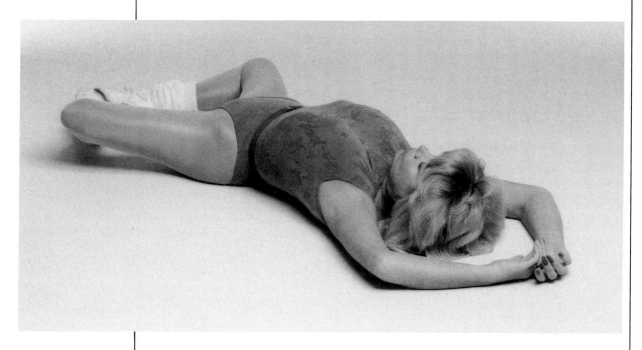

WAIST LINE

Roll over onto your side, taking your body weight on the lower arm and the bottom leg, which should be bent for stability.

Stretch your upper leg out and, lifting your upper arm up and over your head, reach up to the point where the ceiling meets the wall. Hold for a slow count of eight.

Roll over and repeat on the other side.

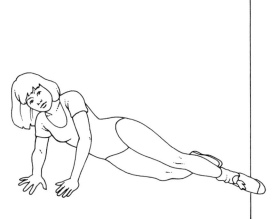

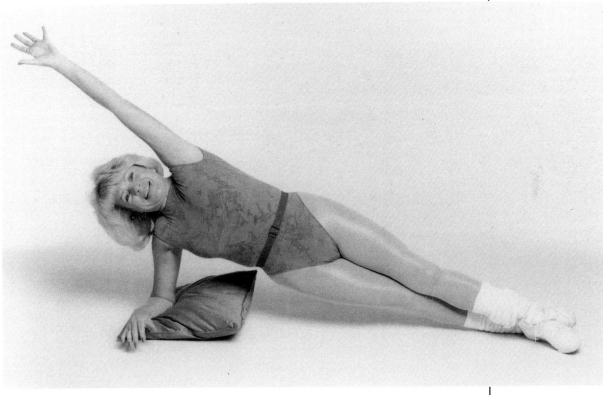

*T*HIGHS (FRONT AND SIDE)

Roll over onto your right side, resting on your upper arm, with the lower leg bent, as you did in the waist stretch.

Grasping your left ankle in your left hand, bring your heel in towards your bottom. Do not pull the heel in too hard. It's not good for the knee. Instead, press out with the foot against your hand, but hold the hand steady so that the foot doesn't move.

Now tilt the pelvis forward and under. You should feel a strong pull down the front of the thigh. Hold it for a count of eight, then shake the leg out, roll over and repeat with the other leg.

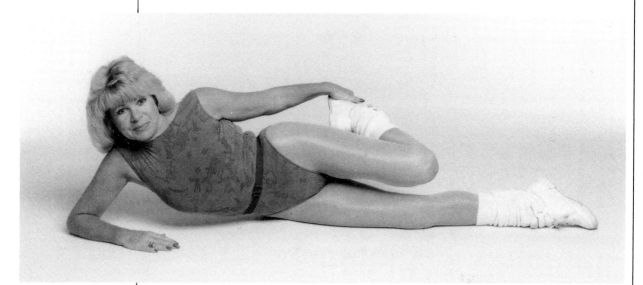

*F*ULL EXTENSION

This exercise is wonderful to do first thing in the morning – it really gets the circulation going.

Still on your back, stretch your arms above your head and reach in opposite directions with the fingers and toes. Stretch as far as you can.

Hold it for a count of eight, then bring your arms down by your sides.

You are now ready for the last, but certainly by no means least, part of your routine – the relaxation session.

CHAPTER 6

RELAX

In the 'good old days' when life was simpler, a person could be born, grow old and die without having travelled more than ten miles outside their native village. Provided Fate didn't deal a wild card like war, famine or pestilence, one could look forward to a reasonably peaceful existence.

Nowadays we live in an age where one can circumnavigate the globe in hours, telephone Timbuctoo in minutes, and have a nervous breakdown in no time at all. Our ears are assailed by traffic and trannies, our eyes (thanks to the miracle of TV) by the latest global disaster, our nostrils by lead pollution and our bodies by acid raid. Is it any wonder that we feel tense?

People try all kinds of solutions in their quest for tranquillity. They eat, drink, smoke, consult psychiatrists and take tranquillisers. Yet we all have the capacity to control our destiny. The power lies within us. All we need to do is learn to relax. The rewards for mastering this life-skill are legion. Relaxation curbs hypertension, aids sleep, eases anxiety, soothes pain. Relaxation can – and will – change your life.

Unfortunately some people have been so tense for so long, they wouldn't know relaxation if it jumped up and bit them on the nose. Check yourself out. Right now. Are you relaxed? Are you sitting comfortably in your chair without a care in the world? Or are you gritting your teeth? Biting your nails? Frowning? Perhaps your shoulders are hunched up round your ears? If so, I bet you didn't even realise you were doing any of these things.

Exercise will relieve stress – temporarily. But for a permanent solution you must learn to let go. And first you need to recognise the relaxation response. Then and only then can you learn to reproduce it: here's how.

Make a fist. Now squeeze your hand tight, tensing up your whole arm. Tight. Tighter. Tightest. Hold for another beat, then let go. That relief you feel flooding through your arm is the relaxation response. Apply it to the rest of your body and pretty soon you will be able to relax in any situation – in a traffic jam, at your desk, or during that crucial meeting. If your body is relaxed your brain will be too. You'll make decisions from a position of power rather than panic.

There are many ways to produce the relaxation response, including yoga and biofeedback techniques. There are also a number of excellent tapes on the market which 'talk you through' the process. I've even made one myself, if you're interested.

Any good exercise routine should feature a few minutes of relaxation after the final stretch. A quiet, contemplative moment to get your life into perspective and collect your thoughts. Once you become more practised you will find that you can unwind anywhere. Below are some simple suggestions to get you started.

Begin by setting the scene. You will presumably already have chosen a time when you know you won't be interrupted, and if you haven't taken the telephone off the hook then please do so now. If it's daylight, draw the curtains. If it's night-time, turn off the lights. Put on your favourite record, something smoochy with a nice even rhythm. Lie down on your duvet, with the pillows arranged to support your head, feet and the small of your back, making yourself as comfortable as you can. I find the 'corpse' position is best, i.e., lying flat with your arms by your sides. But if you have problems with your lower back you may prefer to bring your knees up, keeping your feet flat on the floor. This evens out any arch behind the waist. Now you're ready.

Close your eyes and clear your mind. If this is easier said than done, and your brain keeps hopping round like a Mexican bean then focus on a calm, quiet memory. Alternatively, imagine you are on a desert island, lying on the beach. The sand is warm beneath your body. Run your fingers through the warm sand. Acknowledge the heat of the sun bathing your face in its golden glow. Feel the rays penetrating your very bones. Imagine that a light breeze is blowing in from the sea, fanning your cheeks. Overhead the palm trees are swaying in a cloudless sky. The sound of the surf sings soporifically in your ears and, from somewhere nearby, comes the desultory sound of gulls crying. If you reach out with your right hand, your fingers will curl round a large glass of rum punch. If you stretch out your left, you will come in contact with the companion of your choice. It need not be your current partner. This is *your* fantasy. Who's to know? So indulge yourself and relax.

Begin to breathe deeply. In through the nose. Out through the mouth. Think about your toes. Are they tense? Give them a little wriggle and relax them. Relax your feet (if they're really relaxed they'll drop out to the side).

Relax your ankles, your calves, your knees and your thighs. Tighten up everything inside your pelvis – then relax – let it all go.

Now, starting at the base of your spine and, working right up to the nape of your neck, imagine that each separate little vertebra is dropping down into the floor. Ease the hollow out behind your waist. Lengthen your back. Widen it. Now forget about it. Relax.

Take a deep breath in through your nose, fill your lungs with air, lift your rib-cage up and out to the side. Hold the breath for a second then exhale in a great *whoosh*, driving out all the tension.

Begin breathing regularly again, in at the nose, out through the mouth. Focus your attention on your shoulders. If they're tight, ease them up to your ears, shake them out and relax them.

Relax the top of the arms and the elbows, the bottom of the arms and the wrists. Turn the hands palms upwards and allow the fingers to curl in lightly.

Now concentrate on the neck. If it's tense, and it may well be, (the neck is one of the areas where tension collects with a vengeance), just release it by easing the head gently from side to side. Now centre the head. Feel the weight of it. It's enormously heavy: twelve pounds or so. Imagine that weight falling slowly back through the floor to Australia.

Relax the jaw, let it drop open. Unclamp

the tongue from the roof of your mouth. Relax the eyes – you were probably screwing them up without knowing it – and feel the cheeks softening out.

Draw your eyebrows up towards your hairline, then relax them and feel the tension draining away from the forehead and the scalp. Now imagine that your whole body is heavy and warm, sinking down through the floor, and relax.

With luck – and practice – you should now feel relaxed all over. Your body should feel heavy and warm. Lie there in this semi-somnolent state until the record ends. Don't feel guilty. Enjoy it.

When you've had enough, get up slowly. All your systems will have wound down, and if you spring to your feet you may feel faint or dizzy. Be gentle with yourself. Roll over onto your right side, bring your knees into your chest, put your left hand down and gently ease yourself up into a sitting position. Now stand up. Take a few moments to re-orientate yourself before going about your daily business. I guarantee you will feel like a new person: calm, confident, refreshed and ready to take on the world again.

How long you spend on your relaxation is up to you. Five minutes is generally enough at the end of an exercise routine. But on your exercise day of rest, you might like to spend that available half an hour simply letting go of the worries of the week and preparing yourself for the seven days to come.

Exercise away the frustrations. Relax to relieve the strain. Take responsibility for your own life. Because life, as the song says, is what *you* make it.

CHAPTER 7
LET'S FACE IT

There seems very little point in exercising to retain a taut, youthful body if your chin reveals that you are no longer a spring chicken. Barbara Cartland is reported to have said that you can either keep your face *or* your figure. I believe you can keep both, because the face – dependent though it may be on bones to give it character and expression to give it animation – has a deep-seated muscle structure which can be toned and tightened just as the body can.

Except for certain extreme cases, such as those lined features produced by chronic and consistent over-exposure to sunlight (tan-seekers of both sexes beware) quite dramatic results can be achieved by a combination of exercise, shiatsu pressure-point techniques and massage.

Until recently, the only recourse available to any 'aging primate' (as the over thirties are dubbed by the medical profession) who wished to retain a jowl-free profile, was the ministrations of a competent plastic surgeon. Nowadays even the most expert exponent of the 'nip and tuck' would agree that a face lift which consists of re-structuring loose skin over a firm foundation will look more natural and last longer than one which necessitates shortening already flaccid faschia. The latter technique can only result in some loss of facial range of motion leaving an altogether more artificial expression.

Eva Fraser, who has recently released *Eva Fraser's Facial Workout* on video demonstrates a technique taught her by Eva Hoffman. Fraser claims that ten minutes per day is all that is needed to keep the skin firm and gently reduce incipient sag. Since exercise also encourages circulation, the routine has the added advantage of brightening the complexion and producing a more 'alive' look.

There are, however, a few important points to consider before you begin a facial exercise regime.

a) Don't work-out when you are tired; first thing in the morning is preferable to last thing at night.
b) Make sure that the skin is well lubricated with a good rich cream or an aromatherapy oil.
c) Be careful to breathe regularly and evenly throughout the routine to prevent blood pressure elevation.
d) Practise in front of a mirror for a couple of weeks until you get used to the exercises, after which you can do them anywhere. Working out while watching TV, for example, means you don't have to take time out to do the routine.

Facial exercises are of benefit, whatever your age. Even if you're not at the point where you feel you need them, they are excellent insurance against when you will.

Here are three simple 'tighteners' to get you going.

1 **The Lion** This is a general yoga-based exercise for the face, neck and eyes. For

maximum results you should try to get the tip of your tongue as close as possible to your chin. Sit up straight, with shoulders relaxed and chin parallel to the floor. Breathe in through the nose. Now breathe out, opening the mouth and stretching the tongue out and down. Open the eyes wide and look upwards to the 'third eye' which is situated between the eyebrows. Hold this position, without holding your breathe, for a count of ten. Slowly relax.

2 **Chin Firmer** Begin this exercise as you did the previous one, with shoulders relaxed and chin parallel to the floor. Being careful not to drop the head backwards, tilt the chin up to the point where the ceiling meets the wall. Now relax the jaw so that the mouth drops open. Keeping the top of the head steady, slowly close the mouth again. As you raise the lower jaw you will feel a pull under the chin. This shows the muscles are working. Repeat four times then gently drop the head forward on the chest to relieve any tension on the back of the neck. Finish by bringing the head back to its original position, from which you can begin the third exercise.

3 **Laughter-Line Reducer** Sitting as before, curl the lips in over the teeth and close the mouth so there is no gap between them. Slowly 'smile' pulling the corners of the mouth back towards the ears. Hold the extreme position (but not the breath) for a count of ten, then *slowly* release again.

This last exercise comes from an excellent and comprehensive book by Dr Gloria Klein called *Face-Up*, which also covers Shiatsu facial massage; this is wonderful for dispersing puffiness. The technique, which diverts fluid build-up in the tissues back into the lymph system where it can safely drain away, is too complicated to detail in its entirety; however, here are a few 'pressure points' which you might like to try.

Use the 'balls' of the appropriate digits to apply pressure and, as before, make sure the face is well lubricated before you start. Hold each position for a count of ten and keep breathing.

Place one thumb on top of the other and apply firm pressure to the 'third eye' area.

Press index fingers onto the points halfway between the outer edges of the eyes and the hairline.

Begin by pressing the index fingers firmly into either side of the nose on a level with the inside edges of the eyes and, holding each position for a count of ten, move down half an inch at a time until you reach the outer edges of the mouth.

Tilting the chin up slightly, press the middle fingers into the soft spot behind the ear-lobe.

One further point: the face will always look younger if it is relaxed. A facial massage is an excellent relaxer and has the added advantage of improving skin-tone. My own special guru in this department was a fantastic woman called the Countess Csaky, who had a little place behind the Hilton Hotel and who *did* just about everybody who was anybody. Sadly, she is now retired to Dorset, but her protégé Tai carries on the tradition of excellence which she set.

The Countess is a tiny woman with an impish sense of humour who always wore a white gown and a severe (almost nun-like) head-dress while she was giving treatments. In her late seventies, without a scrap of make-up, she hadn't a line on her face. She was before her time in the use of 'natural' ingredients, her avocado and yeast concoctions being whipped up on the blender while you relaxed under an electric blanket. Her wonderful creams are for sale at the Mayfair Pharmacy and are worth their weight in gold.

One final word. Habitual expressions can often land us with wrinkles we need never have had. If you're deferring getting a pair of glasses because you feel they make you feel older, know that the opposite is the case. Peering at a restaurant menu held six feet from your chest will make you look ancient! And do try not to squint, frown or grimace. Instead, *smile*. Not only is it more pleasant, it does you more good. You see, it takes twice as many facial muscles to grin as it does to glower.

CHAPTER 8
YOU ARE WHAT YOU EAT

Not so long ago, enquiring after free-range eggs or wholemeal bread would have branded you as a nutritional crank – one of *them* rather than one of *us*. The recent salmonella scare changed all that.

The illness – a particularly virulent form of food-poisoning – swept through America and the UK like a mini-plague, leaving considerable carnage in its wake.

This particular salmonella virus had been rife in battery-bred hens and their eggs for years, the felony continually compounded by the feeding of each new generation of birds on the minced-up (and, needless to say, infected) remains of their immediate ancestors. It took a major epidemic, encompassing several hospitals to bring this to the outraged attention of the populace. This forced many farmers to face their responsibilities and destroy their diseased flocks.

Advocates of a return to organic farming, together with ecologically aware groups such as Friends of the Earth, Greenpeace and the Green Party, could have been forgiven for yelling 'I told you so' at the top of their collective voice. Long-time critics of the unacceptable face of Europe's indigenous food industry, they used the free publicity generated by the salmonella episode to hammer home their message. Namely that what we eat, the way we cook food, and the methods used to produce it in the first place, are major contributory factors in the upsurge of such twentieth-century killers as heart disease and cancer.

Prevention is better than cure, is the health lobby's argument, and there would seem to be a great deal of sense in it. By limiting the amount of growth hormones being pumped into farm animals, the amount of pesticides being sprayed on crops and the amount of additives being incorporated into packaged food (to preserve shelf-life and improve colour), they maintain we could at least curtail the escalation of those deadly killers. The incidence of the less serious but still debilitating afflictions of hypertension, migraine, psoriasis, food-allergies, depression and chronic fatigue (ME) could also be reduced.

Health foods, or 'wholefoods', as devotees prefer to call them, are precisely that – the whole food, with nothing taken out. Refined white bread, for instance, is not especially good for you. Wholemeal, on the other hand, with the husk and kernel of the grain intact, provides not only goodness but also essential roughage, which keeps us 'regular' and guards against cancer of the bowel.

One recent survey, carried out in the United States, came to the nauseating conclusion that by the time he reached forty, the average American male is carrying five pounds of undigested meat in his intestines. Such deposits, gathering in pockets in the gut, can lead at the very least to that unpleasant ailment diverticulitis, at the very worst to a colostomy.

The depressing thing is that foods which we have always believed to be healthy, such as eggs, or the humble apple, have latterly proved to be the very opposite. A well-publicised scare in the United States a couple of years ago showed that carcinogens were not only present on the skins of chemically sprayed fruit, but inherent in canned and packaged juices pressed from the apples.

This does not mean that we can never again purchase a supermarket egg or a leg of pork without seriously shortening our lives. It has to be said, though, that a concerted effort on the part of the food-buying public is probably the only thing which will force the food industry, throughout the continent, to put its house in order. However, it does no harm to be vigilant. There are things that one can do immediately to minimise the risks and maximise nutrition without becoming a born-again vegan.

1. Cut your consumption of red meat to one or two servings a week. Hormones, pumped into farm animals, are transferred to the consumer and, although there is as yet no proof that such a build-up of hormone levels will turn you into a male soprano or a bearded lady, better safe than sorry! Substitute chicken (free-range, naturally) or fish or vegetarian alternatives such as cheese, tofu, or pulses (the latter combined with vegetables or grains to give a complete protein).

2. Limit your intake of high-fat dairy foods. A lot of people are unknowingly allergic to them. Instead of soft, creamy cheeses (loaded with fat calories), try quark, goat's or cottage cheese or hard varieties such as parmesan. Drink skimmed or semi-skimmed milk, both of which contain the same amount of bone-building calcium as the full-fat variety. Use water-based spreads. Margarine has the same calorific content as its animal equivalent, butter. What distinguishes the two is the *type* of fat that they are made from. Butter is saturated fat, the kind which, although it may taste good, silts up the arteries. Most soft margarines (not all of them – check the pack) contain poly-unsaturated fats which are more easily assimilated, and don't create a build-up.

For the most healthy fat of all, follow the example of those fortunate enough to live in that area of southern Europe known as the 'olive oil belt'. Olive oil is not only a much healthier cooking medium than the butters and lards of the north, it has a positively therapeutic effect where the arteries are concerned. Tests carried out in Crete showed that, although the general diet was high in fried and fatty foods, the use of olive oil not only decreased the levels of those harmful cholesterols associated with heart disease, it also *increased* those beneficial cholesterols necessary for optimum arterial function.

One dairy food which can be eaten in abundance is yoghourt, not the sickly, sweet, synthetic sort but the thick, creamy natural variety beloved of those remote hill tribes of Asia, so many of whom survive well into their second century. Greek yoghourt makes an excellent substitute for cream on fruit salads and compotes. Live yoghourt is beneficial in replacing active, friendly flora in the gut (vital in the control of unfriendly micro-organisms which, unchecked, proliferate like wildfire), which may have been depleted by long-term use of antibiotics, steroids or the pill.

3. Try, wherever possible, to buy wholegrain staples, stoneground bread, wholewheat pastas, brown rice. These add bulk and all important roughage to the diet. They also provide the right type of carbohydrates (i.e., the sort which fuels energy and keeps hunger at bay) as opposed to the refined variety found in sugar and sugar-based products. Sugar may give an instant 'lift', but it also produces a corresponding 'low', and it breeds the chocoholics and diabetics of the future. Refined carbohydrates provide only empty calories. Wholegrain products fill you up and have a delicious nutty flavour which satisfies at the time of eating and beyond.

4. *Always* wash fruit and vegetables, preferably in boiled water to which has been added a couple of tablespoons of vinegar. This will not only remove any pesticides, it will also take off any trace of heavy metals such as lead. Lead is deposited by car fumes, especially if you buy fresh produce on display in an open air market. Obviously such precautions aren't necessary in the case of fruit which can be peeled, like bananas and oranges.

One other point. Cooking with aluminium pans tends to deposit this other heavy metal in our food during the cooking process. As with lead, the human body is not equipped to cope. Food shouldn't be wrapped for cooking in aluminum foil for precisely the same reason.

5. Take Jane Fonda's advice and 'never eat anything you can't pronounce'. Nobody ever expired from a lack of monosodium glutamate. Scrutinise labels on canned, processed and packaged foods to make sure you know what you're getting. If you're confused, nutritionist Maurice Hanssen's excellent book *E – for Additives*, will inform you about the use and abuse of the now notorious E numbers.

Remember that anything with sucrose, fructose, glucose – any 'ose' in fact – included in the first three of the list of ingredients, is *loaded* with sugar. If you're not worried about your waistline, think about your poor teeth.

Honey, often hailed as a 'miracle' food – along with other bee-associated products such as pollen and Royal Jelly – is simply sugar in disguise. Admittedly, it is delicious stirred into plain yoghourt or spread on hot buttered toast, but there is little evidence to prove the extravagant claims often made for it. It is unlikely that honey lengthens your allotted span, strengthens your immune system or improves your sex life, however enjoyable it is.

6. Restrict your consumption of stimulants. Caffeine is addictive, and can raise the arousal pattern in already stressed individuals to unacceptable levels, triggering complaints such as hypertension, anxiety and phobias. Try the Spanish habit of having a glass of water as a chaser to a strong, black *real* cup of coffee. This is much healthier than consuming endless mugs of instant sludge. Beware decaffeinated coffee too. It's just as acidic as the regular variety, and some of the processes used to leach out the caffeine have been found to produce carcinogens. Herb teas are an acquired taste, but well worth the effort, although they can have differing effects so read the packets to see which are suitable for you. Cinnamon rose, marketed under the Celestial Seasonings label, is particularly delicious.

These few basic guidelines should set you on the path to a healthier eating pattern. The bonus is that this type of diet should stabilise your weight, improve your skin and hair, and limit the possibility of allergic reactions.

The new philosophy of 'Optimum Nutrition' suggests that our food is now so depleted of 'the life force' that we need to supplement our diet with mega-doses of vitamins and minerals. This is not simply to stimulate good health, but also to counteract the positively harmful effects of the chemicals being pumped into our bodies in the name of progress. A well-balanced diet *should* give your body all the nutrients it needs. And indeed man has had to adapt over the ages to environmental changes in order to survive. However, if you have doubts about your vitamin and mineral intake, then a good comprehensive multi-vitamin/mineral tablet taken once a day should keep you on top form.

CHAPTER 9
20 TIPS

How to Stay Slim Without Going On a Diet

Do you ever despair of your expanding waistline? Do you ever say, 'This can't be right. I'm not eating any more than I used to – and yet I'm putting on weight? What's going on?'

What's going on is that as we get older our metabolic rate drops; in other words, the body becomes less efficient at burning up the food we eat as energy (probably because we're not expending as much). We've talked about the metabolic rate earlier in the book, and let's talk about it here again: the message bears repeating.

The energy equation is simple: if you want to lose weight and/or stabilise it, you will have to eat less and exercise more. Why? Because exercise *boosts* the metabolic rate which *becomes lower* when we eat less. This process, first discovered and discussed in detail by Geoffrey Cannon in his book *Dieting Makes You Fat*, is the organism's way of protecting itself in a famine situation, of which dieting is a modified form. In olden days, when long winters or military sieges meant acute shortage of food, the body would drop down a gear so that it needed less fuel to survive. That is why, when you diet, you eventually hit a plateau. The body has simply adjusted its metabolic requirements to the amount of food you are eating.

Now we come to the really rotten bit. When you come off the diet and start to eat normally again, the body doesn't re-adjust itself upwards immediately, so the amount of food which kept your weight stable before will now make you *gain*. That's why it is vital to keep up the exercise routine. Keep working out if you want to slim down your silhouette.

You don't want to become *too* thin, of course. You need a certain amount of body fat to coat the vital organs, and also allow that all-important hormone oestrogen to circulate through the body. It is lack of oestrogen which causes early onset osteoporosis (thinning of the bones) in some ballet dancers and sports people who need to retain a very slim body image. After the menopause, unless you take HRT (hormone replacement therapy), there is a dramatic drop in oestrogen anyway. You need to make sure that what's left has a channel of distribution round the body.

We fifty-years-olds were bright young things in the Twiggy era, when looking any wider than a stick insect was considered positively obese. So we tend to have a rather badly adjusted mental attitude as to what is 'normal' weight. It is no longer fashionable to look like a pre-pubescent starveling.

We have also moved on from the point where losing weight is the prime objective. It's now down to fat/muscle ratios. What do I mean by that? Well, muscle weighs more than fat, so many slim well-toned people are actually *heavier* than their fatter, flabbier counterparts. They are also stronger, and better able to cope with the vicissitudes of life. Keep active, and take a long hard look at your eating habits is my advice. That way you may not even have to go on a diet after all, if you follow these tips.

1. Search the glossy magazines for a picture of the fattest human being you can find. Cut it out. Stick it inside the fridge door. Add an arrow and caption: THIS COULD BE YOU.

2. Say 'No thank you'. No amount of excuses (it's my glands; we're a fat family; I haven't the time to sit down and have a proper meal) or substitutes (appetite suppressants; diet aids; cigarettes) can replace this simple phrase. Trot it out when someone next offers you a second helping of apple crumble, or insists that you order profiteroles because everyone else in the restaurant is pigging out. You are not a pig, you are a person. As such you have the power of positive choice. There is no need to go into long explanations, just 'No thank you'.

3. Throw away your bathroom scales. If you weigh yourself every morning and go into a slump if you've put on half a pound, you're setting yourself up for a miserable day, and one during which you'll probably eat too much to cheer yourself up. Most of us feel we'd be a better, more glamorous person if we could only lose five pounds. But when we've lost that, then what? Will we want to lose another five? And another? Once you get addicted to scale-watching you're in trouble.

4. Try recording what you eat every day for a week. Don't cheat!! Put down every crumb. You'll be amazed at the amount you consume without even knowing it. Also, a pattern will emerge. You'll be able to spot your 'vulnerable' time and do something positive, like going for a jog, to take your mind off it. Mid-afternoon is a favourite time for naughty nibbles, or just before bed. Or you may find you're eating steadily throughout the day and aren't even aware of it: half a slice of bread here, a nibble of cheese there and 'Hey Presto', there's 1,000 extra calories up your shirt.

Recognise your eating pattern and you can start making changes. Be ruthlessly honest though, as it's easy to fool yourself without even realising it. Take the example of the twenty fat people who took part in a recent survey carried out in the United States. They were all having trouble losing weight, so the doctor in charge of their weight-loss programme asked them to note down every morsel they ate for a month. At the end of the month he collected the papers and took the people into his clinic. For the following month, under controlled circumstances, he fed them precisely what they'd written down. And guess what? They all lost weight!

5. Tie a piece of string round your waist. If you don't have a waist, tie a piece of string round the part where your waist ought to be. Make a double knot, so that it is very, very hard to undo the piece of string. Make it snug but not too tight. The next time you eat too much you will feel exceedingly uncomfortable. The string will dig into your too-solid flesh. You'll be surprised how steak and kidney pudding loses its appeal when it produces instant discomfort.

6. Fuel yourself with a good breakfast, then eat a moderate lunch and a light supper. During your long, active day,

you will work off the food you take in in energetic pursuits. If you eat your largest meal late at night, those calories will just lie around in bed with you metamorphosing into fat.

7. When faced with a chocolate gateau, remember Gayelord Hauser's phrase 'This will be a moment in my mouth, three days in my stomach and five years on my hips!'

8. If you begin to bulge as the day wears on, and feel quite bloated by bedtime, then water retention may be your problem. Cutting down on salt could help. Salt absorbs water, and in any case we all eat far more than we need. Most processed foods are loaded with it already, and you probably add more when cooking, so take the saltcellar off the table. If this doesn't help, try a mild herbal diuretic, like Aquaban, or ask your doctor if a prescription for one would be appropriate for you. The drawback with diuretics is that because they flush you out they can deplete the body of mineral salts, especially potassium. A balanced diet should compensate for this but, if in doubt, go back to the daily multi-mineral supplement. If you suffer from cystitis, then diuretics are not a good idea.

9. Try to forget what your mother told you about 'the starving millions': eating up all the food on your plate won't do them the slightest bit of good. If you feel guilty about scraping left-overs into the bin, try to cook less next time, and donate what you save on the housekeeping to a worthy Third World cause.

10. Chew everything twenty times before you swallow it. Some people eat so fast the enzymes in their saliva which begin the digestive process don't get a chance to do their job properly. Result? Dyspepsia. Also, since the stomach takes twenty minutes to register to the brain that it's had enough, you can go on eating long after you're actually full. If you eat more slowly, there's less chance of you consuming more than you need.

11. Always shop after you've eaten, never before. You won't be hungry, so you won't be tempted by those unnecessary items, like double chocolate-chip ice cream, which lighten your purse and overload your waistline. Stock up on nibbles like apples, celery, and carrots. If you don't have cheesecake in the house, you can't eat it.

12. If you have an active social life, don't despair. In a restaurant try to stick to fish and salad, and drink your wine mixed with water. At a home dinner party, try to eat only half of what you're given (three-quarters if the hostess is giving you the evil eye). On no account tell *anyone* you're watching your weight, unless you want to spend the rest of the evening fielding old chestnuts like '*you* don't need to diet' and 'Come on, one little marron glacé won't do any harm'.

13. Be realistic. If you are six foot one and have the sort of pelvis that guaranteed you an easy time in the labour ward, then you will have to resign yourself to the fact that no amount of calorie-cutting or behaviour modification will turn you into Raquel Welch. Even if we lived on lettuce for the rest of our lives most of us wouldn't look as good as Raquel Welch. Keep a sense of proportion: yours. What you should be aiming for is the best version of '*you*' that you can achieve.

14. Try not to feel sorry for yourself. Don't say 'This means I'm never going to

be able to eat another cream bun, fried egg, chip butty.' Never is a long time. Provided you stick to a healthy eating plan *most* of the time, you can allow yourself the occasional slip. Just be extra careful the next day. Most people castigate themselves when they go off the rails, adding guilt to their other problems. Hardly anyone congratulates themselves when they've stuck to their guns. Practise being kind to yourself. Reinforce your efforts now and again with a reward (*not food*) – a trip to the movies, a bunch of flowers, a new pair of frilly knickers. After all, if you don't love yourself nobody else will.

15. Form your own branch of Carboholics Anonymous. If you've had a bad day and the craving for a bar of chocolate becomes unbearable, ring a friend and confess. Confession is good for the soul: it's even better for the hips.

16. If you find yourself wanting to eat while watching TV, realise that you're being manipulated by the medium. Advertising agencies are paid vast sums to make sure you consume the latest pot snack, crisp flavour or ice cream, whether you want it or not. So next time you hear that soupy voice extolling the virtues of something sweet and sticky, operate your power of choice: get up, go into the kitchen, and pour yourself a large Perrier.

17. *Keep exercising.* You know why. But apart from the energy equation, there is a more subtle reason: it will heighten your body awareness. It's hard to focus on 'being good' in November, when the summer holidays seem eons away. However, if you know you have to get into your leotard next Thursday and that *everyone* will *see* you, you'll think twice about that extra muffin.

18. Fibre keeps everything on the move. If you don't eliminate the waste products from your body the residue will seep back into the system and poison it. You will get spots, headaches, piles and bad breath (how glamorous). Nor will you have a flat stomach if it is packed with rotting rubbish. Get rid of it, not with laxatives – they do more harm than good – but by eating more roughage in the form of brown bread and cereals, raw vegetables, baked potatoes and fruit.

19. Egg and grapefruit, bananas and milk, grapes and grapes: the computations are endless. But crash diets have one thing in common: *they don't work.* Even if you lose weight, they don't re-educate your eating habits, so the minute you go off them you'll pile it straight back on again. They're also bad for you in that they deplete the body of vitamins and minerals. Even if your best friend tells you she's just lost ten pounds in three days on peanuts and Pernod (I'm not surprised – her liver probably fell out), don't be tempted. Diet, not diet*ing* is what being fit is all about.

20. Fat creates fat. Need I say more? Cut out as much as you can without making yourself a martyr to boiled potatoes and steamed fish. Replace whole milk with semi-skimmed, use low-fat spreads instead of butter. Put cottage cheese on your baked potato. *Never eat cream.* Opt for low-fat meats like chicken and offal. Learn to love fish. If you succumb to the occasional pork chop be sure to cut off all the crackling. Grill, steam or bake food in a earthenware dish so that it retains its natural juices. Dress salads with yoghourt, herbs and lemon juice. And *throw away your frying pan.*

CHAPTER 10
BASIC BACKS

Almost everyone at sometime in their life suffers from back pain to some degree, from that niggling ache which won't go away to the searing agony of a trapped nerve. Reasons for bad backs vary: bad posture, bad seating, pregnancy, tension, weak stomach muscles. There is even a theory that we were intended to be four-legged creatures, and our spines have never got over the culture shock of finding us defying gravity and standing upright.

As we get older we also have to cope with wear and tear. And since a back, once damaged, is very difficult to put right, it makes good sense to take out insurance against possible problems by developing 'good back behaviour'.

Back trouble which is the result of a slipped disc, osteoporosis (gradual calcification of the bones), a sudden fall or a sporting injury must, of course, be treated by a specialist. But a good deal of back pain can be avoided in the first place by strategic use of simple coping strategies. At the end of the chapter you will find a couple of strengthening exercises plus a couple of stretches specifically designed to keep the back in good working order. If you suffer with nagging back pain, you might like to add them to your daily routine. Remember too that strong stomach muscles 'girdle' and support the back, so keep doing your abdominal exercises.

Before the exercises, here are some tips on back awareness and behaviour modification which will stop occasional discomfort from escalating into permanent pain.

There tend to be two main problem areas where backs are concerned:

a) the neck, shoulders and upper back (cervical and upper thoracic region) where the spine naturally curves out;
b) the area between the waist and the tail-bone (lumbar region) where it naturally curves in.

Let's look at them one at a time.

Neck, Shoulders and Upper Back
The main causes of discomfort here are bad posture (slumping), rounded shoulders and tension produced by sitting in the same position for too long. Those of us most prone to upper back pain are students, writers, VDU operators, housewives (who may go from shelling peas, to washing dishes, to knitting socks – all occupations which call for the back to be slightly rounded and the shoulders hunched forward), and people who, like lorry-drivers or commercial travellers, are forced to drive long distances without a break. Anyone, in fact, who spends protracted periods with their shoulders held in an uncomfortable position is prone to problems.

Raising and angling the shoulders forward leads at best to stiffness triggered by lactic acid build-up in the muscles. At worst it can cause kyphosis, an exaggerated rounding of the upper spine sometimes known as 'dowager's hump'. In post-menopausal women this unsightly affliction is usually the result of oestrogen deficiency, and, with the improvements in Hormone Replacement Therapy is something of which we are thankfully seeing less and less. Amongst the general public, however, it is more likely to happen when the anterior muscles in the front of the shoulder become short and tight through constant stooping. This forces the posterior muscles at the back (since muscles inevitably work in opposition) to lengthen and weaken, to the extent that they are no longer capable of pulling the shoulders up and back into their natural position. The neck then juts forward and the whole weight of the head (anything from 10 to 12 lbs!) ends up hanging from, rather than resting on, the relevant vertebrae. Obviously this puts considerable strain on the neck and shoulder area, and the subsequent localised pain travels upwards to cause tension headaches, migraines and even disturbed vision.

You can guard against all these 'horrors' by taking the following action.

1. If you spend long hours in front of a VDU, make sure your chair is set at the correct height. You should be looking straight at the screen with your chin parallel to the floor. If you aren't, then add a cushion or saw an inch off the legs. Even a fractional tilt of the head can cause strain. On the other hand, why use just any old chair? More and more specialist companies are offering chairs which have been ergonomically designed to give correct support to the spine. The Backstore in Hammersmith stocks a very good selection and offers a delivery service worldwide. You'll find them in the Handy Addresses section at the end of the book.

2. Practise shoulder rolls and the 'three-point pull' (see Warm-Up) regularly *before* tension builds up. (Since fear tends to make one tense the shoulders, this is also a good way of relaxing prior to take-off if you are a nervous air traveller.)

3. Keep the neck mobile. Occasionally drop the chin forward onto your breast bone, or ease it gently from side to side, aiming alternate ears down towards the point of the shoulder (don't raise the shoulder towards the ear). You shouldn't drop the head back, though, as this hyper-extends the neck. Above all, don't roll the head in a complete circle (especially at speed) since this will cause the vertebrae to grind together.

4. No matter how pressing the task in hand, give yourself a break every couple of hours. Concentration flags at this point anyway. Stand up and have a good stretch. If you're driving, stop at the next service station and have a cup of tea. If you regularly use a special piece of music for the relaxation phase of your workout, you might like to transfer it to tape and play it in your car if you know you're going to be driving a long distance. Pop it on when you start to feel the strain. You'll be amazed how you react; because the brain will have begun to associate that particular piece of music with calmness and tranquillity, you will respond to it immediately. By turning it on you can radically alter your state. Just make sure it's not something that sends you to sleep!

5. At the end of a hard day, get a friend or your partner to give your neck and shoulders a gentle massage. They should begin by pressing the balls of the thumbs into the base of the skull (on either side of the spine). From there progress down

and out towards the points of the shoulders, holding the pressure at each point for 5 seconds and moving the thumbs about an inch further apart each time. It's amazing just how much tension this area can hold, and the release of knotted muscles by a little loving manipulation can be absolute bliss.

6. Try not to resort to pain-killers. They deaden the sensation but don't attack the root problem, with the result that you can carry on regardless and damage the back even further. This also applies to the other area under discussion.

The Lower Back or Lumbar Region
The main causes of problems here are bad posture again (take the individual with a beer belly as an example; all that extra weight pulls the spine into an exaggerated and unsightly curve), pregnancy (for roughly the same reason), force of gravity, carrying shopping or a heavy briefcase in one hand (or wearing a shoulder-bag on the same shoulder all the time), lifting heavy weights by bending from the waist with straight legs, sitting badly in ill-designed chairs.

Here's how to cope.

1. *Beer belly* Cut down on beer, obviously. The extra weight on the front of the body is not only unsightly, it can actually pull the lower back into a position known as lordosis. If beer is not the problem (lordosis can be hereditary), then a strong network of abdominal muscles will flatten the stomach, support the back and improve the posture. Excess curvature in the lower back can also be caused by tight erector spinae muscles (the big interlocking set of muscles that runs down the entire back on either side of the spine). Do the stretch for the lower back (given in the flexibility section) often. You can even do it sitting upright (while watching TV, for instance). Just make sure your back is well supported, and hug the knees into the chest for a while.

2. *Pregnancy* Most of us are past this; however, some of us never get rid of that lower back discomfort which starts when the weight of the baby begins to pull the back out of alignment. The 'pelvic tilt', invented by Lotte Berk, is wonderful for relieving this. Lie supine, knees bent, feet flat on the floor. Roll the spine out slightly to create a hollow just big enough for you to slide your hands under. Now take the hands away and do the opposite. Pull the back down, pressing it into the floor and tilt the pelvis up. You can do this to good effect even if the closest you've ever been to being pregnant is assisting at the conception! It is an excellent method for keeping the spine mobile and preventing the vertebrae from becoming impacted.

3. *Force of gravity* As mentioned before, the head can weigh up to a stone. Balanced on top of the spine, this weight – coupled with the force of gravity which presses us earthwards – can squeeze the discs together, causing discomfort. Practise the pelvic tilt frequently to alleviate this.

4. *Shopping/briefcases/shoulder-bags* Distribute weight evenly between both hands (shopping); carry your briefcase or bag on a different side each day.

5. *Lifting* Always squat, never bend over. Hug the object close to the chest and stand up, using the muscles of the thigh and bottom to push you upright. The same thing applies if the car conks

out, or you are moving a piece of heavy furniture from one place to another. Never 'put your back *into* it' otherwise you will put your back *out*. Stand with your back to the car/sofa, which will then support it, and use the strength of your thighs to press the body (and the object) backwards.

6. *Chairs* We've already covered this in the first section, but remember, it doesn't matter how well designed the furniture is if you don't use it properly. Whether you're typing, driving or simply relaxing, make sure you always tuck your lower back right into the base of the seat. Driving creates spinal shock (for the same reason that horse-riders often get bad backs – all that bouncing up and down), the severity of which depends on the state of the roads, the speed you are travelling and the condition of your shock absorbers. You can now buy beaded seat covers which absorb a lot of the shock and give your spine and the back of your legs a massage at the same time.

Make sure your work station is well out of draughts and be very careful when executing any movement which involves lifting and twisting at the same time.

Your back is tremendously strong but, as with anything in this life, it will repay you according to how you treat it. Give it a little tender loving care and it will never let you down.

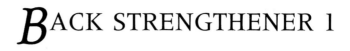BACK STRENGTHENER 1

Lie down in a sphinx position, taking the weight of the upper body on your lower arms. Don't force the arch in your back. Don't raise the eyes towards the ceiling. Don't lift the pelvis off the floor. This is a fully supported lower back extension. You'll normally feel a stretch in the stomach.

If you feel any discomfort in the lower back, bend the elbows and bring the chest a little closer to the floor, increasing the curve over a period of time as your lower back becomes less tight.

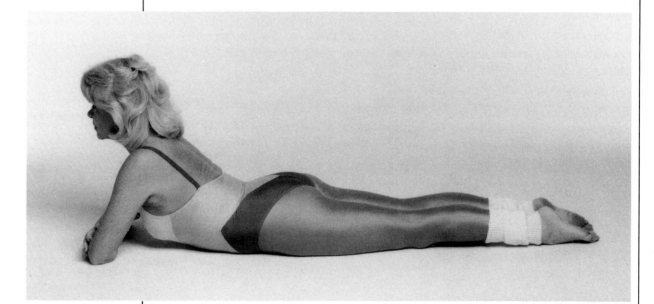

BACK STRETCH 1

Begin on hands and knees, hands under the points of the shoulders, knees hip-width apart. Sit back between the feet, easing the lower back down towards the floor. Stretch the hands out ahead, pressing down with the inside of the upper arms and the breast-bone to extend the stretch into the upper back and across the shoulders.

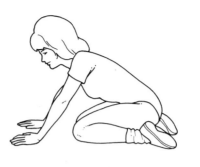

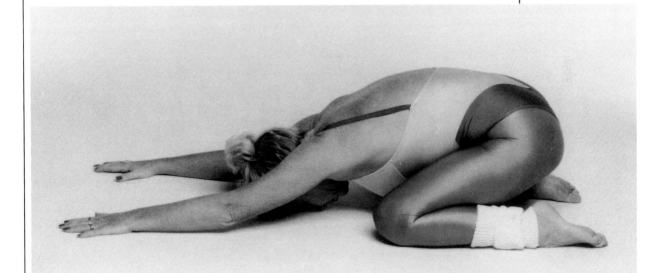

Hold this position for a slow count of eight, then relax.

BACK STRENGTHENER 2

This exercise will strengthen the upper and lower back simultaneously.

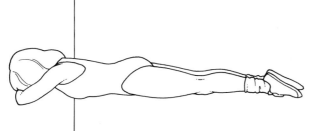

Lie face down with the forehead resting on the hands. Now raise your right arm, your left leg and your head slowly off the floor. As with the previous exercise, don't exaggerate the curve of the lower back. However do try to stretch the limbs out as much as possible. Hold for a count of four, breathing regularly.

Relax and repeat with the left arm and the right leg.

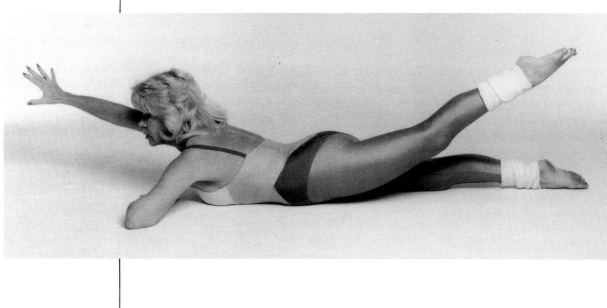

BACK STRETCH 2

Sit up straight with one leg stretched along the floor and the other hugged in close to your chest. Flex the toes of the stretched leg.

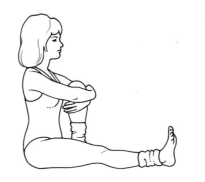

Now, lift the body up and over the thigh, feeling the spine elongating.

Reach across your stretched leg aiming the tips of your fingers towards the toes of the flexed foot. Keep the arm parallel to the leg.

Breathe in through the nose and, as you breathe out, reach forward another inch.

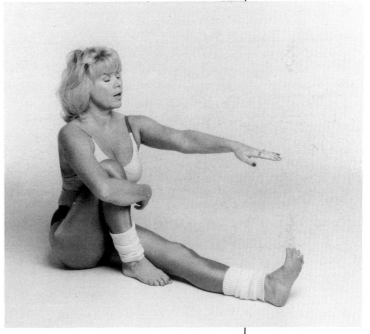

CHAPTER 11
A WORD ABOUT POSTURE

Maintaining the back in prime condition is all very well, but if in between exercises you stand like a sack of potatoes you might as well not bother. Posture: that's what it's all about. And if that good old-fashioned word conjures up pictures of pigeon chests and ramrod backs, think again. For not only does posture affect our body image, in that clothes hang much better from an upright frame, it also affects other people's conception of and attitude to us. A person who slouches gives out untidy, uncaring signals and if we don't care about ourselves, how can we expect other people to care about us? Our body image is the clue to who we are. It doesn't necessarily follow that if we are slovenly of body, we are slothful of mind, but it can certainly give that impression.

Although it may seem like an oversimplification, our physical appearance can also radically alter our mental state. So why not alter it for the better? Let me explain. If you are depressed how do you walk, stand, behave? My guess would be that you slump, slouch and curl in on yourself as though the world were a big bad place of which you were expecting the worst. And if you anticipate the worst, that's exactly what you'll get. By altering the physical position of your body, by standing up and looking the world in the eye, you can often alleviate the depression that got you slouching in the first place. You will feel more in control of yourself, and the world will become a much more amenable place as a result.

Try this. Stand up now. Tell yourself you feel strong, in control, self-reliant: *believe* it. Now look at yourself in the mirror and smile. How do you look? Confident? In charge? Of course you do.

Now allow your shoulders to droop, your stomach to bag, your knees to sag. Let your mouth fall into a disconsolate mode. How do you look now? How do you *feel*? How do you think you would look to anyone else? Which of the images looks the more youthful, vibrant, alive? Which of the images makes the best impression? Exactly.

Begin with your posture. Stand tall. Standing tall will make you look slimmer.

The trouble is, if you ask someone to stand tall, their natural reaction is to tense up, throw their shoulders back, and stick out their chest; this exaggerates the curve in the lower spine, and causing them to stick their behind out for balance.

How do you achieve a natural, relaxed and elegant stance instead? Well, the old Victorian remedy of the book on the head is hard to beat. To keep a book balanced that way, the neck and spine have to be in perfect alignment, and the chin needs to be held parallel to the floor. Think of the fluid grace of those African women who daily walk miles with huge pots of water or bundles of washing on their heads. Think of their long lissome necks and the way their limbs move. They almost look as though they were attached to Heaven by, yes, you guessed it, an invisible piece of string.

Make that piece of string work for you. Instead of standing up, imagine that you are hanging down like a puppet, with the string attached to the top of your head. Imagine that the force of gravity is sucking you down towards the ground and that you are swinging gently in the breeze with your feet just grazing the floor.

Feel your shoulders dropping away from your head. Feel the consequent lengthening in your neck. Feel your pelvis dropping away from your rib-cage, and the consequent lengthening of your back. Pull your stomach in and up under that rib-cage. Tuck it out of sight. Now feel the arms dropping away from the shoulders, the hands and fingers relaxed at the end of fluid wrists. Feel the weight of the feet (still swinging just above the ground) lengthening the legs, easing any tension out of the knees and ankles. Swing there for a minute, quite relaxed, focusing on the rhythm of your breathing. Then begin to walk around the room, trying to retain that feeling of relaxed mobility.

Practice in front of a mirror every now and then until your mind gets used to the feeling of what you look like when your posture is good. Pretty soon, if you are in a situation where you know you are beginning to stand badly, you'll only have to say 'strings', quietly to yourself, and your body will 'assume the position' by reflex action. The better you stand, the better you look, the better you feel.

And now, one last look at that African woman with the pot on her head. What has she got on her feet? Precisely: nothing. Now I'm not suggesting that you shoot off to the office or the Supermarket au nature, but if you are female and usually wear 6-inch heels, then do your feet and your back a favour and adopt a more sensible mode of footwear. There are some gloriously pretty flat shoes on the market, and trainers are just about *de rigueur* with sportswear. Although stilettos may add length to the leg, they also tip the body forward, which means you have to arch the back to keep yourself from falling flat on your face. A moderate heel is fine, but anything more than an inch and a half will show. No matter how sexy you think they are, high heels create sore feet, which show in your expression.

To sum up: the complete works of William Shakespeare on top, comfortable shoes on the bottom, and 'strings' in the middle. These three Ss (Shakespeare, shoes and string) will work wonders for your posture, just as the other three Ss (strength, stamina and suppleness) will for your constitution. All you have to do is stick at it until it becomes part of your life style.

CHAPTER 12
EXERCISES TO AVOID

Much as I hate to be negative, there are times when you have to say 'no'. There follows a list of exercises which you should never do, under any circumstances. So that you don't think I'm being dictatorial for its own sake, I am including the biological reasons why.

If you are a jogger, a squash player or a home exerciser, then don't be tempted to include any of these exercises in your routine. If you go to an exercise class locally or belong to an amateur rugby or football team where all or any of these – now contra-indicated – moves are taught as part of the training routine, then it might be better if you changed your class, or your coach.

Over the past ten years, more in-depth research into how the body functions has been conducted in laboratories worldwide than took place over the whole of the previous century. As a result, many of our beliefs as to what is safe exercise and what isn't have been completely revolutionised. Some of the physical jerks, such as toe-touching and straight-leg sit ups – encouraged by physical education coaches in the past – have since proved to be less than appropriate.

Unfortunately education is failing to keep pace with the rapidity of the research, and at times the information takes rather longer to filter down to the exercising public than it should. The result is that some quite unnecessary injuries are still being caused by well-meaning but ill-informed instructors. Nobody goes out of their way deliberately to harm a client, but exercise is very definitely one area where the 'what was good enough for my father . . .' attitude simply has no place.

The old attitudes of 'no pain – no gain' and 'going for the burn' have thankfully been discredited for some time. Since you get out of it what you put in, you should always feel like you are having to make an effort when you are exercising. The body needs to be challenged to do a little better if we are to see improvements in our muscle tone and cardio-vascular fitness; but pain is always the body's way of saying *enough*.

Listen to your body. When in doubt, leave it out. About the following exercises you need not have even a shadow of a doubt: avoid them like the plague. *You have been warned!*

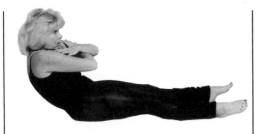

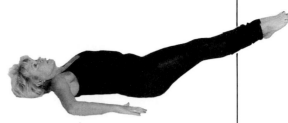

STRAIGHT-LEG SIT-UPS

At one time sit-ups were thought to strengthen the stomach muscles: they don't. Instead they work the hip flexors, which run from the lower spine to the top of the legs. Although some hip flexor work is necessary, over-strengthening leads to arching of the lower back and can exacerbate any tendency to lordosis. Add to that the fact that unconditioned people, attempting to haul their upper body weight up this way, tend to push their stomach out, causing a pot belly, and you will see why this exercise is inadvisable. Marching, cycling or jogging are good ways to strengthen the hip flexors. Curl-ups with bent knees are the safe way to a flat stomach.

DOUBLE LEG RAISES

This exercise is the same thing in reverse. It also strengthens the hip flexors. The stomach muscles only contract in self-defence (or rather in defence of the lumbar-sacral spine, which is put under pressure by the weight of the legs 'hanging' on it), so there is minimal conditioning. This exercise also produces considerable internal strain, and can cause compression injuries to discs and vertebrae, as well as tears to muscles or damage to ligaments. No matter what an instructor using this exercise says, it is *impossible* to keep the back flat while doing double-leg raises: don't even try.

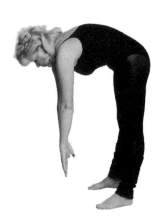

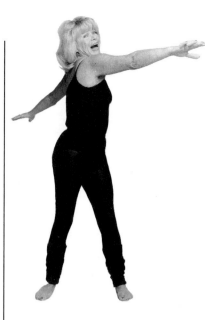

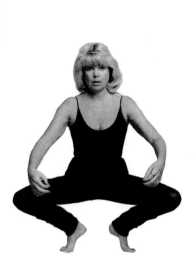

TOE-TOUCHES

Exercise, Stop, Danger, a publication of the British-Australian Fitness Leader Network, claims that this is 'the most dangerous exercise in the world'. This is because flopping forward with straight legs to touch the toes puts tremendous hydrostatic pressure on the lumbar discs. Bouncing down only makes things worse since, apart from potential danger to the spine, you may also tear the hamstrings, which run down the back of the thigh, or extensor muscles of the lower back, both of which this exercise is supposed to stretch. To add insult to injury, (or vice versa) the exercise creates a condition of total body tension. And since muscles can only be stretched safely when they are relaxed (and there are other, more appropriate exercises which *do* stretch the hamstrings and lower back), there seems to be no valid reason for doing it.

SPINAL TWISTS

Rapid spinal twisting should always be avoided, as it may damage the intervertebral discs and lead on to severe back pain. Clearly, twisting is a movement which is included in the normal range of motion, but any exercise designed to facilitate such movement should be slow and controlled, and/or done in a position where the back is supported by the floor.

DEEP KNEE BENDS

Although bending the knees is essential for safe lifting techniques (see Chapter 10 Basic Backs), the feet should always be placed hip-width apart and under the knee itself. If the feet are kept together then the knees will be hyper-flexed, allowing the unsupported body weight to hang on the kneecap. This can cause injury to the ligaments, muscles, tendons and even cartilage. For the same reason – even if the feet are placed correctly – you should be careful never to bring your thighs lower than parallel to the floor.

CHAPTER 13
ROUTINE RUN-DOWN

Clearly the days mentioned here are only my suggestions – you can begin on any day you like!

MONDAY, WEDNESDAY, FRIDAY	TUESDAY, THURSDAY, SATURDAY
Warm-up: 5 minutes.	Warm-up: 5 minutes.
Aerobics: (walking, swimming, cycling or exercises) 20 minutes.	Calesthenics: (Tums, bums and legs, plus backs – if you have problems there) 20 minutes.
Cool-down stretch: 5 minutes.	Cool-down stretch: 5 minutes.
Relaxation: as long as you like.	Relaxation: as long as you like.

SUNDAY
Twenty minutes' blissful relaxation: optional, but *very* worthwhile.

If you have an area, such as the stomach, which is your particular bête noir, you can include 5 minutes extra on your aerobic days just to work on it.

Be consistent; little and often is the best policy. Think of it as being an investment in yourself. However, if you do happen to miss a day, don't succumb to guilt or despair and give up entirely. Just begin again the next day as if nothing had happened. Remember too that you shouldn't push yourself to carry on if you are ill, especially if you have a virus; your body needs all its reserves to make you well again. The good thing is that since exercise stimulates the immune system, you should be less ill, less often.

Expect to *feel* results in two to three weeks; expect to *see* results within six.

PART TWO
LIFE STYLE MANAGEMENT

CHAPTER 14
HOLISTIC HEALTH

It's all very well getting your body into shape, but what about your mind? Fitness is more than lissome limbs and a regular resting heart rate. Attitude also has its part to play in being fit at fifty. The things that are important are: stress control, a sound eating plan (as opposed to sporadic dieting), enough sleep, regular medical check-ups, cutting down on mood-altering drugs (including alcohol), and keeping an open mind. All these things come under the new heading of holistic health. It is important to see the organism i.e., you, as a whole rather than a series of fragmented parts.

It's no longer enough to do a bit of running, give up cigarettes and expect that to see us through to a productive old age. Rather we must realise that all areas of our physical and mental well-being are interrelated. With that in mind, here are a few suggestions to help you develop that harmonious balance which is the *true* measure of good health.

Rediscover the forgotten art of conversation; people who work on machines (assembly line, word processor or computer) and then go home to watch TV can find themselves alienated from the rest of the human race. They forget how to communicate and become withdrawn and unhappy. Try joining a club (debating, drama or dinner) where you will be forced to flex your conversational muscles and make friends in the process.

Reward yourself. If you do a good job, treat yourself to a small reward like a trip to the movies. Be sensible: don't buy a box of chocolates if you've just lost 5lbs on a diet. But don't put yourself in a double-bind situation either. If you reach your target – whether it be weight or work – don't tell yourself you could have done better. Likewise, if you don't reach your target, don't say you couldn't have done worse. Either way you lose. So where's the incentive?

Rehearse your way to success: practise 'the inner game'. Sports-people use this all the time mentally to plan their strategy in advance, but the concept can easily be adapted to an everyday situation. If you're facing something which you dread, like a difficult job interview or a meeting with an irate bank manager, talk yourself through it. Imagine the worst possible scenario. Confront it and cope with it in your head. When you get to the real thing it'll be a lot less horrendous than you imagined and, like Baden-Powell and the scouts, you'll 'be prepared'.

Rework your philosophies. An outmoded attitude like 'I'm too old for that' will make you old, whatever age you are. Let your hair down now and again. Eat ice cream in the street, stay up to see the sunrise (even if you *do* have to get up for work in the morning), play cricket with your young nephew. Don't stand on your dignity. There will be plenty of time for that when you are pushing a hundred.

Regain your confidence. Master a new skill; children do this all the time but, once we've left full-time education, we very often stagnate. Attempt something that's a real challenge. Learn to swim or sky-dive, or even fly! The joy of discovering you still have the ability to absorb knowledge will give you the confidence to keep adding to your expertise. Life is a learning process, and with each new challenge you broaden your horizons, your self-confidence and your circle of acquaintances.

Revamp your exercise routine, if you have one, that is. If you're bored to death with your work-out class, change it. Exercise is useless if you don't enjoy it. If you've been doing aerobics for ages, try something quite different like California stretch. If you've been exercising outdoors, work inside for a change. If you've been into one-to-one competitive sports like squash, try a team game.

Rekindle romance. If your current liaison has become a bit dull, don't abandon it out of hand. Inject a little pizzazz instead, with a weekend by the sea or candles, music and a home-cooked meal or perhaps a relaxing massage with scented oils. Whatever the state of your bank balance, there is something you can do to show you care. The results will be commensurate with the effort, not the expense.

Remain in control. Re-think your eating habits. Cut down the triggers that send you heading for the cookie jar. Only eat in one place in the house. Don't consume food on the move, while cooking or when watching TV. Cut out between-meal snacks, limit your alcohol intake, and say no to seconds. That way you'll stay trim without having to diet at all.

Re-open dialogues with long-forgotten friends. Go through your old address book and drop a postcard to all those people with whom you've lost touch over the past decade.

Reacquaint yourself with the rest of the world. Don't be too set in your ways. If you always buy the same paper, take one with a totally opposing political viewpoint for a change. Open your mind to the other side's ideas. If you get CNN on Satellite Telly, take in America's notion of World News; you'll find it quite different to Europe's. Take a night-school or linguaphone course in French or German. Don't be insulated and you won't be isolated.

Rearrange your schedule. Too much to do, too little time? Don't scurry from one job to another, never finishing anything properly. Make a list. Put the most important task (or the one you don't want to do the most) at the top and tackle that first. Cancel out anything you don't have to do. Be ruthless – especially if your list is heavy on things you promised to do for other people.

Repeat this philosophy at least once a day. 'I'm okay. Not perfect, but okay. My opinions are as valid as the next person's.' This is called 'self-talk'; and it works, particularly if you lack self-esteem. Pretty soon you'll start believing in your own worth. Then you'll stop apologising for yourself.

Resuscitate your bank balance: Go through your investments and discard any that haven't given you a return of at least 10% in the last year. Scan the money pages for the best pension options. Review and renew if necessary. Check that your house insurance is adequate and up to date. Make sure your life assurance will assure your nearest and dearest of a decent life style should the worst happen. Make a will. Money isn't everything, but security becomes doubly important in the fifth decade.

Revise your attitude to others. Regardless of what you might think, people in general are pretty pleasant. They'd rather do you a good turn than a bad one, especially if you're nice to them. If someone is being nasty to you, don't snap back; smile. At best it'll defuse the situation, at worst it'll take the wind out of their sails.

Retrain yourself. If you've fallen into bad habits, like constantly moaning, never being in time for dinner or saying 'no' to your teenage son as a matter of course, interrupt the pattern. Just because you've always done it doesn't mean you always have to.

Repeat three times a day: the past does not represent the future. Because you once failed at something (playing tennis, cooking choux pastry, learning Russian dancing) doesn't mean you'll always fail. You may not have been ready for it before. Believe in yourself, and have another go. You might be in for a big surprise. If you fail again, who cares? At least you gave it your best shot.

Relax. Make use of your leisure time doing something you want to do, like going to the movies or the theatre, seeing friends in a café with a bottle of wine, or just going to bed early with a cup of cocoa, a Pavarotti record and a pile of magazines. Bliss! If you're a workaholic who spends free time looking for more work to do, this may be difficult. Keep trying: it gets easier as you go along. (See chapter 6.)

Resolve that from now on you'll be positive. Open yourself to new experiences; say 'yes' rather than 'I don't think I can'. Life is short, and when you're fifty you can't afford to waste a minute being miserable, or indecisive or just plain boring.

CHAPTER 15
STRESS

Stress has been with us since the stone-age. But it's only in the last twenty years that it has been recognised as the psychological trigger for many physiological ills.

Mid-life brings its own special crises: loss of libido, intimations of mortality, marriage problems which suddenly emerge when the children eventually leave home, and husband and wife discover that they seem to have little left in common.

Lack of communication can see a marriage spiralling down to a level where separation or divorce become inevitable, largely because of stress overload. This chapter will help you take greater control of the stress factors in your life.

Not all stress is bad for us, of course, and we all need a certain amount. We each have an Optimum Stress Level, where just the right amount is expected of us so that we can give of our best. This kind of stress is enjoyable, stimulating.

Positive and negative stress are different things altogether. Positive stress occurs when life-demands exceed our capabilities. Whatever the cause, it is when these demands push us over the hump of the human function curve and down the other side that stress becomes distress and the problems begin. We wake in the night, dry-mouthed and with pounding heart. We lose our temper at the slightest thing, jump every time the phone rings and either stuff ourselves with fast food or lose our apetite completely. We become accident-prone, forgetful, disorganised: we can't cope.

When stone-age man was faced with a life-threatening situation, his body would become flooded with nor-adrenaline – the 'fight or flight' hormone. His system assumed a war-footing, and fats, pumped into his bloodstream, gave him that extra burst of energy to tackle or retreat from his adversary. This gearing up process was reversed once the extra hormone had been utilised in combat or retreat. The body then relaxed back to its pre-stimulated state.

Fortunately space-age man (or woman) seldom finds himself in a true life or death dilemma, but the twentieth-century body has not yet learned to modify its reactions to perceived danger. It cannot tell the difference between a marauding mammoth and a report that should have been in yesterday. Nor-adrenaline poured into the system is seldom used up, and undissipated fats left lurking in the blood are laid down as cholesterol; this silts up the arteries and causes heart problems.

Negative stress is caused when we are underused. It attacks those with boring, repetitive jobs such as assembly line workers or women trapped at home with the housework. Lack of stimulation, both mental and physical, leads to a depressive cycle which can wind down into apathetic despair.

So what can we do to harness the destructive power of stress and make it work for rather than against us? First we need to find our Optimum Stress Level, which is unique. Some thrive on round the world travel, hotel living and incipient jet-lag. Others break out in a cold sweat at the thought of having to find a parking space on a weekly shopping trip. The trick is to know your limits and to stay within them. Recognise situations that you know will trigger stress, and either avoid them or nip patterned reflexes in the bud before they gain the upper hand. Prevention, rather than cure, is the order of the day.

Here are some coping strategies to get you started. A word of advice: try to make changes one at a time. Too many drastic alterations all at once will simply add one more area of stress to your life. Long-standing habits are difficult to break. So use a little psychology on yourself: pick the easiest problem and deal with that first. Your success will then motivate you to tackle the harder options.

COPING STRATEGIES FOR POSITIVE STRESS

1. Try not to bring work home. Change to leisure mode as soon as you leave your place of employment. Remind yourself that the most successful people are not those who work the longest hours, but those who have learned to organise, delegate and leave themselves plenty of free space in their lives. Ask yourself what, apart from meeting the debts, you are working for? Don't get into the 'golden handcuff' situation where your possessions begin to own you rather than the other way round. Maybe you're using work as an excuse not to have to communicate with your husband/wife/significant other? If it's to lay down a good pension, remind yourself that if you don't slow down, you may never live to enjoy it!

2. Relax. I know, I keep harping on about it, but it is important. Buy a relaxation tape and play it in the car on the way home. Enrol in a yoga class. Get a bio-feedback machine. Listen to soothing music. Getting irritated may be just a habit you've fallen into. Take control by saying 'Nothing has the power to irritate me unless I give it permission'.

3. Indulge in a series of short weekend breaks once every three months rather than one long, summer holiday. Often a change of scene is enough to bring back a sense of perspective.

4. Make sure you do communicate with your other half, if you have one. There is no greater buffer or hedge against the slings and arrow of the world, than a loving shoulder on which to cry or a sympathetic ear in which to pour your troubles. If relations have got to the point where the pair of you are barely speaking, then make an effort, however small, to improve things. A bunch of flowers, or a pair of silk boxer shorts, will work wonders. A surprise visit to a restaurant or movie is another great ice-breaker.

5. Eat regular, wholesome meals.

6. Get eight hours' sleep a night, if you need it.

7. Do aerobic exercise to use up the nor-adrenaline residue and stop it turning to acid and ulcers. Avoid competitive sports such as squash: they simply add to your arousal level. Team games are okay since the buzz of victory or defeat – both equal on the stress scale – is spread amongst a group.

8. Before going into a stress situation, such as a presentation or an after-dinner

speech, take three really deep breaths to calm yourself down.

9. Lay off artificial stimulants (coffee).

10. Try a little time-management. Don't allow things to pile up. Never let a piece of paper pass through your hands twice; answer mail as soon as it arrives with a card, a short note or a phone call.

COPING STRATEGIES FOR NEGATIVE STRESS

1. Don't hang around the house counting your wrinkles or filling your face with food. Go out, though not shopping. Buying things you don't want is a fruitless and expensive way to fill the gap in an empty life. Take in a matinée, go for a long walk by the river, have a picnic. If you're short of cash, visit the public library, pick up a good book and read all the latest magazines for free.

2. Make yourself useful. If the kids have gone and your nurturing skills are going begging, offer them to a deserving charity. Time is more precious than gold when it comes to helping out the disadvantaged, the sick, the needy. Meals on wheels, the Oxfam Shop, the Samaritans – They can all do with an extra pair of hands. Charity work is very rewarding, and if you need to feel needed, then it's just the ticket. It will take your mind off whatever troubles you may have, and widen your social circle at the same time. If you don't know where to start, call your local council for information.

3. Get a job. The number of school leavers is dropping and there are at least some jobs around. If you haven't worked for years and are terrified of the prospect of going out in the marketplace, remind yourself that if you can organise a family, you can organise a business. And think of the money – money means independence.

4. Retrain. Explore the possibility of a local authority grant for mature students and get yourself some qualifications. Try to go to college rather than studying at home, because getting out and joining in the extra-curricular activities is half the fun. Otherwise there's the Open University, the Open College or the University of the Third Age. They all do summer schools where you can meet up with tutors and fellow students once a year at least.

5. Eat regular, wholesome meals.

6. Get eight hours' sleep a night, but no more; depressives tend to sleep too much to try to block out the world. If you find you're sleeping in excess of ten hours a night, buy an alarm clock and *use* it.

7. Join a leisure club, or a local authority work-out class. This will make you look better, feel better and make friends.

8. Turn a hobby into a business. If you're a great cook, a good knitter or if you've always wanted to be a writer, now's the time to turn your talents into cash. Cater parties, machine knit plain sweaters in glorious wools, join a writer's circle and get on with it.

9. Lay off depressants, including alcohol.

10. If the day stretches ahead of you, bleak and empty, don't turn on the TV and give up on life: participate instead. And try to face each morning with the expectation of good things to come. Anticipate the best. Your attitude to life governs what you get out of it. As Shakespeare said, 'There's nothing either good or bad but thinking makes it so.'

CHAPTER 16
SWEET DREAMS

Shakespeare also wrote (and I paraphrase) that sleep knits up the ravelled sleeve of care. How true – for without sleep life unravels with a vengeance. Too little of this precious commodity sags the skin, makes us ill-tempered, ruins our concentration and exposes us to every prowling germ or virus.

Recent research at Harvard and the University of Texas has shown that those old wives' tales about a 'good night's sleep' are soundly based in fact; sleep is a healer. Clinical tests now prove that there is a biochemical link between deep sleep and a strong immune system; simple bed-rest can have quite a dramatic therapeutic effect, especially in cases of viral infections such as flu.

Those elements in our system which trigger deep, dreamless sleep (unlike REM – rapid eye movement – sleep which is associated *with* dreams) also help recharge the body's defence mechanisms. Both triggers begin in the gut, where bacteria produce compounds known as muramyl peptides (so potent that a millionth of a gram can add several *hours* to a night's sleep). On reaching the brain, the muramyl peptides set off the production of interleukins, which in turn stimulate lymphocytes (the immune system's defensive cells), which then go on to tackle and destroy invading, harmful bacterias.

The basic message here is clear: sleep is good for what ails you. How much sleep, though? There is no recognisable norm. Some individuals are lively as crickets on four hours a night; others feel washed out on less than nine.

This brings us to insomniacs, those unfortunates who find the balm of a restful night as elusive as the pot of gold at the end of the rainbow. How can you cope if you are one of those? Don't hop on the see-saw of sleepers at night, and pep-pills to pull you through the chemical hang-over next morning. Pills are not only addictive, they're counter-productive. The system becomes used to them quite quickly, so that an ever-increasing dose is required to gain the same effect. Worse, they repress the aforementioned REM and cause extreme depression, since our dream-time is the period during which we subconsciously get to grips with our daytime problems.

Here are some other 'nos' if you want to encourage a visit from the Sandman.

Cut out coffee, if not completely then at least after 8.00 p.m. Don't take strenuous exercise in the evening – it will wind you up rather than calm you down. Remember that alcohol is not only a depressant but a dehydratant. A drink before bedtime will lead you to wake in the wee, small hours beset with nameless fears and fancies. If you *do* have the occasional one too many then two pints of water drunk before you go to bed, will counteract the pre-dawn horrors.

Conversely, here are some positive coping strategies to send you off to the Land of Nod.

1. Other than last thing at night, *do* keep up the exercise routine. Regular exercise is one of the greatest promoters of sound sleep. Programme your workout for earlier in the day. This will ensure that the body is free of any lurking nor-adrenaline, and that you are physically pleasantly tired when bed-time rolls around.

2. Practise the simple relaxation techniques dealt with earlier in the book. Once mastered they will trigger the body into sleep-mode as soon as you slip between the sheets.

3. Try a warm, milky drink such as Horlicks or Ovaltine (the low-cal version if you're worried about your waistline). Milk contains tryptophan, a sleep-inducing amino acid. If you can't tolerate milk then camomile tea can be similarly soothing.

4. Get into the habit of going to bed at the same time every night. This will programme the body to expect sleep.

5. Read for a few moments, something heavy and boring – like the telephone directory. Don't watch TV.

6. If a daytime problem persists in making your brain behave like a record that's stuck in a groove, get up and write it down. It's amazing how committing something to paper prevents it cluttering up the cranium.

7. Make sure your bed is comfortable. It seems obvious, but often a change of mattress, the addition of a duvet or a self-indulgent hot-water bottle are all that is needed to turn a night-time thrasher into a sound sleeper.

8. Are you woken early by dawn light? Invest in thick, lined curtains. Otherwise those little masks which many international airliners give out are miraculous. If traffic noise is a problem, then use ear-plugs or even double-glaze the house, depending on which your budget dictates.

9. Finally – try not to worry. Often the anxiety produced by thinking you won't go to sleep is enough to ensure that you don't. Who knows, maybe you're one of the lucky ones who only need four hours a night. Use the time you gain to write a bestseller!

CHAPTER 17
HOW TO CHOOSE A CLASS

This book is not intended to be the be-all and end-all of your exercising life. I hope it will get you interested enough eventually to take you out of the house and into either a sport or an exercise class.

I genuinely believe that there is no one in this world, no matter how over-weight or out of condition, who would not benefit from a well-run, well-supervised class aimed at their age and level of fitness. I emphasise the 'well-run', however.

Exercise is the true elixir of life. It shouldn't be an ordeal, it shouldn't leave you gasping for breath or dizzy or puce in the face. A certain amount of muscle stiffness is to be expected in the begin-ning, especially if the most strenuous thing you've done in the past ten years is curl up in front of the telly with a Mars Bar. It should not be unbearable, though, and it should never persist past the third week. You should never suffer any pain in the joints, either during or after a class. If you do, while working out, stop immediately.

Here is what to look for when choos-ing an exercise class.

1. It should be reasonably small, with fifteen to twenty people at most, de-pending on the size of the room. No teacher can oversee more than this at one time. Nor can she get to know her pupils individually, which she needs to do if you are to get the most out of your efforts. Everyone is built differently.

Their capabilities are different, and so are their potential fitness levels. If the room is packed to the gills and there isn't space to breathe, let alone move, then you can safely surmise that you are in the hands of someone more interested in their pro-fit than your health. Of course there's nothing reprehensible about making a profit, just so long as it's not at your expense.

2. The room in which you work should be warm and well-ventilated, and have a sprung floor to cushion the impact on your joints if you are doing any form of aerobic work. There should be a loo and a supply of drinking water nearby and preferably – though this is a luxury rather than a necessity – showers.

3. The music should be appropriate: live-ly and stimulating for the up-beat part of the class, smooth and relaxing for cool-downs and relaxation. It should have an even beat with no pauses or tempo changes, and it shouldn't be so loud that it damages your eardrums.

4. Class should begin with a good warm-up to limber up the body and get the juices flowing. It should finish with a cool-down period. This is very impor-tant, since it minimises post-exercise stiffness, not to mention the fact that if you go out sweaty and hot, no matter how warm the day, you will catch a chill. Also, if the class has done its work well, it will have triggered off the natural

adrenalin in your body, leaving you pleasantly 'high'. Without a cool-down you run the risk of leaping into the car and wrapping yourself round the nearest lamp post.

5. Last, but most important, your teacher should be trained. If in doubt, ask her. Unless she's got something to hide she'll be happy to tell you her qualifications. She should have a thorough knowledge of basic anatomy and should make sure, before she admits you to her class, that you have no medical problems or old injuries that might be exacerbated by the exercises. She should be enthusiastic about her subject and be able to impart that enthusiasm to other people. She should give instructions in a clear audible voice, be open to questions and ready with informative and easily understood answers. She should treat each member of the class as an individual and have a mental file which covers their abilities, their vulnerabilities and their future possibilities. If she doesn't know your name by the third week, she doesn't know her job. She should encourage rather than criticise. No one should be bullied into making an effort beyond their capabilities or be embarrassed before their peers. Only a bad teacher has to resort to these methods to get the best out of her class. Finally, your teacher should be in good shape herself, living proof that the exercises she teaches, work.

You may live in an area where your only option is the weekly keep-fit class at the local church hall. However, if you are spoilt for choice and don't know where to start picking your way through the movement maze, here are some brief explanations of the contents of various classes currently on offer in fitness centres nationwide.

I've taken the liberty of grading them for their appropriateness for the over fifties. *R* stands for recommended, *HR* for highly recommended and *NR* for not recommended. *NR* does not mean that the class is not appropriate for other age groups. In all cases I have erred on the side of caution.

HIGH-IMPACT (OR FAST) AEROBICS (HIA) *NR*

Variations on fast, running on the spot movements using mainly the major muscle groups of the lower body (behind and legs). To be effective the work-out must raise the training heart rate and keep it raised for a minimum of twenty minutes. Can be very challenging and hard on the joints and pelvic floor. Proper shoes *must* be worn. Well-organised centres offer a choice of beginners, intermediate and advanced.

LOW-IMPACT AEROBICS (LIA) *HR*

Large, travelling movements taken at a much slower pace than high-impact, and incorporating a good deal of upper body work (arm and shoulder) to keep the training heart rate up. Kinder on the joints and very effective as a means of fat-burning. Note: classes need to be kept small to allow for larger movements.

BODY CONDITIONING *R*

May involve an element of aerobic work or simply consist of muscle-toning and stretching. (Depends on the teacher's interpretation). Tightens up the wobbly bits.

LIA WEIGHTS *R*

A modified, low-impact class using light (1lb) handweights during the aerobic section and ankleweights (2lbs) during the floor exercises. Good for balancing upper and lower body.

NEW BODY *NR*

Faster version of LIA Weights class, using longer, more challenging aerobic section and no ankle-weights.

STRETCH AND TONE *HR*

Rhythmic limbering-up exercises designed to stretch and strengthen the whole body. No aerobic element, so they need to be augmented by swimming or a walking programme for overall fitness.

SKI-FIT *R* (if you're a skier)

Series of progressive classes (usually lasting from six to twelve weeks) designed to minimise on-piste stiffness, strengthen sport-specific muscles and help you make the most of your two-week break. Some aerobics may be included, but usually not.

CIRCUIT TRAINING *R* (if you work at your own pace)

A workout which can be as challenging as you want it to be. The exercise area is set out in a number of 'stations' each one of which the participant visits during the course of the class, which can last anything from twenty minutes to an hour. Stations alternate between cardiovascular work (stair-stepping, rebounding, skipping) and resistance training, (which itself alternates between upper and lower body conditioning to allow the mus-

cles ample recovery time between sets). The participant works as hard as his or her personal fitness level allows at each station for a set period of time (usually thirty to forty-five seconds) then moves on. A super circuit involves doing two complete rotations of the room. To improve you need to do more, in the set time, at each session. Some abdominal work is always incorporated in the routine. Good for men.

JAZZ *NR*

Show-bizzy, dance-based class which involves complicated routines. Though enjoyable, a background in professional dance or at least a brilliant natural rhythm are needed to get the most for your money. Not recommended for anyone with two left feet.

CARDIO-FUNK *NR*

Lively, funky, young class based on modern rhythms and sounds. Go if being surrounded by gyrating teenagers doesn't make you feel like Rip Van Winkle.

BALLET *NR*

Slow, disciplined, elegant class generally conducted to classical music. Most classes are aimed at children, but dance centres in larger towns offer some mixed adult classes. Very relaxing if you're supple, hard work if you're not, and nostalgic if you did it as a child.

BELLY DANCING *R*

Great fun and guaranteed to make you a wow at the office party.

TAP *HR*

A chance to let off steam and make a lot of noise. Wonderfully therapeutic and suitable for all age-groups.

YOGA *R*

Calming for mind and body, yoga is not an easy option. Some of the recommended positions take years of practice to perfect. Involves excellent beneficial breathing techniques, and may include dietary recommendations. Devotees report lessening of tension and a feeling of being at one with the Universe. Music, if used, tends to be esoteric and relies heavily on the sitar.

WATER AEROBICS *HR*

Excellent even if you can't swim, since classes are invariably held in the shallow end. Suitable for anyone, of any age and any condition (except those who suffer from cystitis) since the water not only cushions the body but provides resistance against which the muscles have to work. Good value. Good fun. Check water is comfortably warm, that instructor is qualified in this particular method, and that there is always a lifeguard on hand.

TAI CHI *HR*

Based on the ancient Chinese mind and body discipline, Tai Chi is practised en masse by factory workers all over China. A series of slow controlled moves requiring a great deal of concentration and commitment, it is excellent for improving balance and co-ordination. No music.

AWARENESS THROUGH MOVEMENT (ATM) *HR*

Floor-supported exercise, done without music, based on the theories of Russian Israeli physicist, engineer and martial arts expert, Moshe Feldenkrais. Classes aim to take the body back to the pre-learning stage of childhood and re-educate the central nervous system in correct usage. Feldenkrais believed that bad postural habits, learned early and practised over many years, are what cause most of the aches and pains experienced in later life.

WOMAN'S SELF-DEFENCE *HR*

Absolutely vital in these days of escalating crime. Classes usually run for a set period (six weeks) and will give you some really useful tips on how to get out of trouble should the worst come to the worst. Good to know that brain rather than brawn is what is needed to come unscathed out of a handbag- or even life-threatening situation. If these classes do nothing more than help you not to look like a victim, they're well worth it.

RELAXATION *HR*

Gentle exercises to help you release, or stop the build-up of, tension, and to teach you the relaxation response. Won't get rid of your spare tyre. Will help you sleep, alleviate stress and stop you worrying about it (the spare tyre).

THE STEP *NR*

The latest craze from the States, this is a very strenuous class in which all exercises are conducted on and around a step that can be adjusted (height-wise) to suit your particular fitness level. So a world-class athlete could work stepping up and down on a twelve-inch-high step and holding 10lb hand-weights, while a sixty-year-old could do the same routine alongside but working on an inch step without weights. Gives a good cardio-vascular work-out, and is much kinder to the joints than HIA since the stepping movement exerts only the same force as walking at 4 m.p.h. while giving the same results as running 7 m.p.h. Based on old army bench-step routines, The Step can be very effective. Drawbacks are that it can be boring, hard (whatever they say) on the knees and it tends to build up muscle bulk on the thighs and bottom.

Once you've chosen your class, how do you make the most of it?

1. Be honest. Teachers, no matter how well-trained or professional, are not miracle workers, nor mind-readers. So if on arrival your teacher asks you whether you have any problems that she should know about and you don't tell her about your dodgy knee (for fear she'll say you cannot join in) and five minutes into the warm-up you twist it, then you have no one to blame but yourself.

A good teacher knows how to give you a good work-out *without* damaging that knee. She will advise you to avoid certain movements and keep an eye on you to make sure that you do.

2. Be sensible. If she doesn't ask you about possible problems, and you have asthma or suffer from diabetes or epilepsy, or if you have high blood pressure, a history of heart disease in the family, lower back problems or are taking special medication, then you *must* volunteer the information. You should also check with your doctor whether you should be doing a class at all. It's your duty to yourself to take responsibility for your own body.

3. Be self-centred. Once class begins, concentrate on yourself, not the person next to you. Whether they do fewer or more repetitions than you is immaterial. Work at your own pace so that *you* gain maximum benefit. Class is not a competition. Of course you don't want to let yourself down and look like a wimp, that's only natural. But nor do you want to be crippled forty-eight hours later. Whatever you do, *don't* work through pain of any sort. If it hurts now it will hurt tomorrow. Remember, your teacher cannot feel what you feel. She can judge what she thinks you are capable of, but she is not you. If you can't keep up, then don't try, especially if you're doing aerobics. As a general rule you should be able to talk to the person next to you quite comfortably whilst raising your heart rate. Try singing along to the music (quietly if you're the shy type). That way you won't be able to hold your breath.

Similarly with stretching. Don't look at your neighbour and expect to be able to do whatever they're doing. They may have been coming to class for ages or just be naturally supple. The rule of thumb here is that it takes about three months of regular exercise to stretch a body out.

4. Be prepared. If you have no option but to join a general class and you attend regularly, there will inevitably come a time when you feel you can do it all. No matter how good your teacher is, or how often she changes her tapes or routines, there are only so many exercises and variations on same. At this juncture,

motivation is all. If you feel you're not improving, boredom may set in, enthusiasm wane and you'll find yourself making excuses not to turn up. Fight the temptation. If you succumb, your body won't thank you for it. There are several ways you can step up your training level if you wish to do so.

5. Be flexible.
a) Buy a tape and work out at home between sessions.
b) Cross train. Go swimming, jogging or buy a bike.
c) Wear ankle weights (2lbs) and wrist weights (1lb) in class during the body conditioning sections. The extra loading will make your muscles work harder with corresponding benefits. Don't make the mistake of thinking the heavier the weight, the more the benefit. Heavy weights build heavy muscles; light weights streamline them. Note: never wear weights during warm-up, high impact aerobics or stretch periods. If you can't get weights locally you can buy them mail-order from Carita House; the address and telephone number are in the Handy Addresses section of the book. They also stock attractive exercise wear.

6. Be regular. To make the most of your exercise class you should 'make it a date'. An occasional missed session does no harm (nobody's perfect), but if you only roll up once in a blue moon you're wasting your time, energy and hard-earned cash.

CHAPTER 18
THE ICING ON THE GINGERBREAD

Being fit at fifty has more to it than a strong heart and a healthy diet. It's also about being happy with yourself. It's about being confident that you're looking, as well as feeling, your best. It's about making the most of what you've got, once you've got it.

This is not vanity: it's simple common sense. First impressions are important, and the sad fact is that the way we look has a great deal to do with the way we're treated by other people. Everyone wants to be loved, and it's not frippery or foolishness to make the best of your assets. Being glamorous, having style, élan, whatever you want to call it, does not mean you have cotton wool between your ears.

Looking good is not an indulgence: it's a duty. Lank hair and unkempt shoes will give people the impression you don't care for yourself. And if you don't care, why should they? You don't have to be vain or self-indulgent to look good. You don't need oodles of money or unlimited time. You just need to be organised.

1. **Wardrobe** Most people's wardrobes could do with a good sort out. Practically everyone has things hanging in the back that they will never wear again. Mistakes, impulse buys, items that just aren't your colour. *Weed them out*. It's amazing how cathartic a good spring-clean can be. Dump everything you haven't worn for two years. Try on what's left. Throw out anything that doesn't make you look good, at your present weight with no make-up and your hair uncoiffed. This is a tall order. You'll probably be left with not very much, but what is there will be a firm basis on which to build.

Bundle up all your rejects. Sort them into piles. Good stuff can go to a second-hand shop. Something which looks frightful on you could look sensational on someone else and you'll make a few pennies into the bargain. Anything else that is clean and undamaged can go to Oxfam or the local Scout Jumble Sale. Anything tatty or torn or beyond repair should go in the bin. Get rid of everything straight away. Before you change your mind. Be particularly ruthless with shoes. Shoes date faster than anything else.

Lay out what's left and have a look at it. Make a list of what you need to buy to update it. An extra blouse and a few well-chosen scarves and pieces of costume jewellery can transform a wardrobe. New shoes in the latest shape may be all that's needed to pull an 80s outfit into the 90s. Set aside anything that needs cleaning, and have it cleaned. Make another pile of what needs mending, and don't hang it up until it's done. Keep a sewing kit by the ironing board so you can replace those buttons on-the-spot, before you put things away.

Start to invest in shoe trees, padded hangers, classic items such as cashmere and silk. There is no need to break the bank. A new cashmere every winter (get them in the sale), another silk shirt every summer, will soon build up to a respectable wardrobe. Get a good coat. With our climate it's probably the item you'll wear most. Budget for one good piece of clothing per season, something which will fit in with what you've already got. Start with a jacket and build slacks and skirts around it. Get the best quality cut and cloth that you can afford. After a certain age one should aim to look classy, not trendy. Cheap and cheerful gear is out, with one exception. Buy tracksuits from chain stores and change into them as soon as you come home. This simple expedient will lengthen the life of your 'good' clothes, stop them seating and bagging and save on cleaning bills.

2. **Image** If you really are hopeless with clothes and don't know where to start, you might like to invest in a session with an image-consultant. This will set you back about £50, but could save you making expensive mistakes on future shopping trips. An image consultant will be able to advise you on your style (classic, glamorous, tailored, frilly) and show you how to make the most of your own particular shape through clever camouflage. If you have a small bust and a big behind, for example, then a skin-tight sweater under a dirndl skirt will only emphasise these points. A slim skirt (not tight) and a jacket with padded shoulders, on the other hand will balance out your silhouette.

3. **Colour-coding** Similar to the above, but working on the colours that suit you. There are several companies around (Colour Me Beautiful, The House of Colour) who will give you a consultation and advise you on what shades to go for and/or avoid. Fees are similar to those for image consulting and in both cases, you will usually be given a handy little reference diary as an *aide-memoire* on shopping trips. Colour-coding is based on skin tones. If you have gold-based skin, for example you should avoid shades with blue tones (both for clothes and make-up). The opposite applies if your skin has a blue base. Colours that clash can make you look harsh or jaded, those that tone, enhance your natural colouring and give you a glow. As a refinement, certain types look better in bright or muted colours. If you don't have a colour consultant in your area, or can't afford to invest in a personal session, Colour Me Beautiful do a series of books which explain the principles of colour and image in more depth. They also sell mail-order make-up to suit your skin type.

4. **The body beautiful** Whatever clothes you wear or colours you choose, if the body underneath the garment is saggy you will end up looking like a sack of potatoes. Use the information at the beginning of this book to get into shape, and you will look great in an old pair of jeans and your husband's cast-off cricket sweater. If motivation is a problem, set yourself a goal. On the first of April, buy yourself a new swimsuit. Put it on and stand in front of a full-length mirror. If you don't like what you see, you have three months to do something about it. Once in shape, try not to backslide. Britt Ekland has said in print that she never likes to be more than three days away from perfect. A good maxim. If you are always in reasonable shape then you can forget the big panic when you get a sudden, unexpected invitation. Once the body is there, pamper it. Set aside a certain time every week to do all the things you need to do (nails, hair, bath,

face, washing, ironing, shoe cleaning, repairs) to keep yourself and your image in optimum condition. Sunday afternoon is a good time. Get everything done that you can and then forget about it for the rest of the week.

5. The extras

a) *Nails*. Short, long, brittle or strong, nails need to be clean. Give yourself a manicure once a week. If there isn't time during your Sunday routine, do them while you're watching your favourite television programme. Give them at least half an hour to dry. Do your toenails at the same time. If your nails are short, wear a muted colour, if they're long and strong, flaunt them in a bright vibrant shade. Choose a lipstick that matches your skin and a varnish to tone, rather than the other way around. Buy the best quality you can and always wear a base coat. Matt varnish looks classier than glossy, and doesn't chip as easily. Always wear rubber gloves for washing up and gardening gloves for weeding: prevention is easier than repair.

b) *Teeth*. Bad teeth can ruin a whole face. In these days of improved nutrition, fluoride and cosmetic dentistry there's really no excuse for them. If they're dingy, you can have them 'bonded' with a lighter, decay-resistant coating. If they're chipped or crooked you can have them capped. Bridges will fill out gaps and stop what is left from becoming loose and falling out. I am assuming that you clean and floss your teeth regularly. Now that we're into Europe, take a leaf from the continental's book and learn to use a toothpick properly (there's an art to it). It's also a good idea to make an appointment with a dental hygienist to have your teeth professionally cleaned every three months. Often it's gum disease, rather than bad teeth which is the cause of multiple extractions and dentures in later life.

c) *Eyes*. Nothing is as aging as peering at a menu from a distance of two feet. It is much better to get a decent pair of glasses. There are some wonderfully flattering ones on the market, as well as contact lenses in both hard and soft varieties. You can get glasses with coloured or graded lenses and disposable contacts that you put in for a week and then discard. You can even get tinted contact lenses. Glasses should be a fashion accessory, worn with a flourish rather than taken out surreptitiously and perched on the bridge of the nose while no one's looking.

After the age of forty eye muscles get tired and vision becomes less acute. There are exercises you can do to re-activate the muscles. If you have the time or the patience to do them then there is an excellent book on the subject by W.H. Bates, which you'll find in the Further Reading section at the end of the book.

d) *Hair*. You can be wearing the latest creation by Yves Saint Laurent, but if your hair's tatty it won't work. It can be a mistake to chop your hair off as you get older. A swinging mane of shiny, conditioned, well-trimmed hair says young at any age. If you can't afford a weekly appointment then a good cut by the best hairdresser in town followed by a regular six-week trim (make your next appointment before you leave the shop and put it in your diary as soon as you get home) is the least you can get away with. Wash your hair frequently *before* it looks like it needs it – and condition, condition, condition.

Colour depends on you. Highlights round the face can give a real lift, but if you're very dark, give streaks a miss as the strong contrast will make you look grey. Avoid anything too harsh; jet black, bright red and glaring yellow will make you look like a superannuated punk. If you go for an all-over colour remember that it's expensive to keep up; coloured hair needs plenty of conditioning, and nothing looks tackier than black roots. Never have a colour *and* a perm, as this will damage your hair.

6. **Face** If you can't run to a regular monthly facial, at least give yourself a weekly face-pack in the bath while you read the Sunday papers. Make sure you choose one which is suitable for your skin type. There are packs for dry or oily skin, packs to close open pores, and brighten up a dull complexion. If cash is a problem then you can find cheap and efficient natural ingredients in your kitchen. The yolk of an egg, applied with a pastry brush, lubricates dry skins. The white, put on the same way, dries up excess oil. Be careful to wash both types of mask off with cold water unless you want the egg to cook on your face! For the acne-prone, plain yoghourt is pleasantly soothing. And don't throw away your old tea-bags. Dampened with cool water and placed over the eyes while you are relaxing for your regulation twenty minutes, they will banish any puffiness and bring back the sparkle. Herb tea bags are even better, particularly camomile. Cold mint tea bags, stroked over the face and neck, make an excellent substitute for face tonic. Invest, if you can, in a good exfoliating agent. Skin becomes less efficient at sloughing off the dead outer cells as time goes on. A gentle facial scrub will push the business on.

So far as make-up is concerned, less is more when you pass fifty. By all means

keep abreast of the trends but don't be a slave to fashion, and don't get stuck in a time-warp either. If you're still wearing false eyelashes and white lipstick then clearly it's time you updated your image! Don't wear bright blue eyeshadow, bright red lipstick, base that's darker than your skin tone (especially if it ends in a line at your chin) or powder, which collects in and emphasises incipient wrinkles. Unless you have a very greasy skin, a foundation with a hint of shine gives a more youthful glow to your face than a thicker, matt one. Never go to bed with your make-up on. Always wear blusher, but be sure to blend it in well. If you've really no idea how to apply make-up you might like to take a lesson. This should not be from someone with a vested interest like the cosmetic salesperson at your local departmental store, but somewhere like Joan Price's Face Place, or at your local Beauty Salon. Here you can experiment discreetly in the privacy of your own cubicle. Absorb the information that works for you and discard the rest. Find your own style, don't slavishly adopt someone else's.

7. **Check-up** An annual medical check-up is very good insurance. If you are a member of BUPA they have all the facilities to give you a thorough going over. If not, your local Well-Woman clinic should cover most things. At the very least you should get a regular mammogram and smear and, if you are taking HRT (hormone replacement therapy) you should have your blood pressure tested every six months. If you have access to one of the all-too-few machines available in this country it's also a good idea to get a bone scan.

CHAPTER 19
TREATS

Whether it's hereditary, socially in-grained, or part of our genetic make-up, women spend a great deal of their lives nurturing other people. We also have a sense of guilt about indulging ourselves. Years of putting the kid's school shoes before our new dress, or missing a trip to the cinema to make sure the boss's letters get out on time have left us with the feeling that money or time spent solely on ourselves is some-how not on. This is nonsense.

Our generation spearheaded the idea of the equal woman. We did the ground-work that has given the young women of today the freedom they have. Yet no matter how self-possessed and in control we appear to be, because we were brought up pre-women's lib, the brain-washing which was passed on to us still lurks in our psyche. Those codes of ethics which insisted that a man came first, that a woman's role was to make sacrifices, are difficult to get rid of.

Fifty is the age to lay those untruths to rest once and for all. Now's the time to tell yourself — and believe it — that there is nothing reprehensible about enjoying yourself, being self-indulgent and saying 'me first'. Men do it all the time, after all.

1. **Outings** Whether you have an in-terest in music, art, Shakespeare, an-tiques, rock 'n roll, or foreign travel, now's the time to follow it up. Join the local Theatre Society. This will give you access to advance notice and booking facilities (at concessionary rates) for coming productions, plus social events linked to the theatre, like tea with the cast or tours backstage. Art galleries usually run similar schemes where you get invitations to preview exhibitions before they are thrown open to the general public. Get the paper each week and check what's on at the movies, and go. If your partner isn't interested (or you haven't got one at present) don't be deterred. These are treats for *you*. Rope in a girlfriend or, be daring, and go alone during the afternoon. Visit stately homes or gardens. Join the National Trust. Check your local bus company for day trips. Like Londoners who've never been to the Tower of London, we're usually woefully ignorant about the wonderful sites and scenery in our own back yard. Listen to your local radio station and scan your paper for information on forthcoming concerts close by or a little further afield.

If it will interest, intrigue, inform or just plain amuse you, *do it*. If you live in the south of England, go to France on a day-trip. If not, try a long weekend by the sea. Sea air is wonderfully bracing even in the winter. Take loads of books and a warm coat for beach-side walks to blow the cobwebs away. Many hotel chains offer special deals, as do British Rail.

2. **Individual indulgences** Have a sauna, to clear out your skin; a facial to keep wrinkles at bay and deep cleanse your face; a massage — with aromather-

apy oils – totally luxurious; a new hair-do, to go with the new you. Have an hour in a flotation tank – it will clear your mind. Have lunch by the river, or in a country pub. Choose somewhere with a wonderful atmosphere (log fires, gleaming horse brasses, friendly service) and/or a fantastic view. Book ahead to make sure you get a good table. Order your favourite food and watch the world go by. Soak up the atmosphere, listen to other people's conversations. If you're alone, *don't* take a book; be confident in yourself. At home, go to bed early with a quarter-bottle of pink champagne, a plate of creamy scrambled eggs and the latest bestseller.

3. **Collective treats** Have any of the above, but in quantity. Drop subtle hints around your birthday or Christmas time; a ten-session voucher will make the big day last for three months.

One of the best days I've ever had was when my now teenage son was eighteen months old. I was trying to look after him and the house and (during nap times and after he'd gone to bed), finish the third part of a science fiction trilogy on a tight deadline. It was a cold, rainy February that year and I was exhausted, bad tempered, and totally strung out. My husband, either in self-defence or out of the kindness of his heart – I've never worked out which – booked me a day at The Sanctuary in Covent Garden. For an all-in price I entered a world of leather loungers, Caribbean warmth and para-keets on perches beside a pool where carp swam. I had a sauna, a massage, a swim, a health food lunch, a jacuzzi and a sunbed.

That day, I want to tell you, was better than a fortnight's holiday. Most beauty salons do a day of treats at a special price.

If you book one, make sure that as well as the usual massage, facial and sunbed, you choose a few totally frivolous treatments. Have your legs waxed, your eyebrows plucked, your toenails painted. Life would be very empty if this was all you had to do with your time, but now and then being pampered and cosseted can make you feel like a new person.

4. **Health farms** Champneys, Inglewood, Stobo Castle, Ragdale Hall: these are the names that dreams are made of. Get away from the madding crowd and allow yourself to be the centre of attention for a change. You can go for a weekend, a week or (if you've won the pools) ten days. Health farms are not cheap – especially when you consider you may be living on lettuce leaves – but if you calculate that there are none of the usual extras associated with a summer or ski-ing holiday, then the prices hold up against any reasonably luxurious package.

If it's out of the question as an extra, a visit to a health farm can make a wonderful alternative to the usual annual sun and sand package holiday. On arrival you will be weighed and measured and given a diet (anything from total starvation to gourmet health food) and allocated four daily treatments (mud baths, G5 massage, that sort of thing) which are included in the price; if you want to add more treatments they cost extra, so be warned. There is usually a heated swimming pool and a selection of exercise classes, and you may be able to golf or sky-dive or go on long, group walks. Your bedroom will be comfortable, with television and a bath or shower en-suite but no telephone, the inference being that you are there to get away from the rat-race. There are no fax machines or mobile phones or transistor radios.

Health farms are usually located in old country houses in the centre of beautiful gardens which feed the spirit as well as the eye. They are centrally heated and self-contained, so that in mid-winter they give you the sense of being concooned against the world. Their effect can be quite miraculous: you may go in looking grey and flaky, but you will come out glowing, invigorated and probably half a stone lighter. If nothing else they're worth it for the peace and quiet.

CHAPTER 20
DON'T BE ALONE OUT THERE

Loneliness is one of the blights of the late twentieth century, which is a curious paradox. With more people on the planet than ever before, it becomes increasingly difficult to make contact, at any age. At fifty plus it can seem almost impossible. There are Over Fifties Clubs, of course, but these tend to be aimed at the older, staider end of the market. Women, unlike men, cannot hang around in bars without giving the wrong impression. Adverts in lonely heart's columns tend to turn up some very strange responses. So, if you are a single career girl, a divorcee, or simply someone whose children have recently left home, where do you go to find convivial company and prove to yourself and everyone else that there's plenty of life left in you yet?

1. **Make contact** Don't sit by the telephone expecting people to get in touch with you; they have their own lives to live. Friendships need to be worked at, or they will simply shrivel away. *You* pick up the phone and make that call. At least people will be reminded that you're about, so next time they're looking for a fourth at bridge or are throwing a Hallowe'en party, your name has more chance of coming up. Remember too that there are people older and lonelier than you.

How long is it since you wrote a letter – to anyone? Instead of slumping in front of the TV feeling neglected, flip through your address book and drop a line to faraway friends. Never mind if you haven't made contact for ages. If you only write one letter a week, you'll have contacted fifty-two people by this time next year. Even if only half of them write back (you must allow for people having moved on) you can expect upwards of twenty-five letters: you'll have opened up your world.

2. **Work out** Join an Exercise Club, not just for the benefit of your body but also of your social life. Clubs are a great place to meet members of the opposite sex while getting fit. Sign up for an appropriate class. Class members tend to congregate in the canteen or the bar afterwards. If a posh facility is beyond your pocket then consider local authority Leisure Centres. Some of them are quite spectacular and, since they are heavily subsidised, the fees are nominal. While you're there look on the notice board for special offers, sports clubs in the area, ideas to expand your social circle. Mixed sex sports to get involved in are orienteering, or any racquet game (join your local tennis club/squash league). If you're interested in running or cycling, don't be solitary, join a group where you can go on excursions with a crowd. You're bound to meet new faces at lunch or in the pub afterwards.

3. **Have fun** If you are a thwarted thespian why not join the local Amateur Dramatic or Operatic Society? Societies usually rehearse during the winter sea-

114

son and normally put on a pantomime and/or a spring production. Rehearsals are an entertainment in themselves, and a great way to get a free night out of the house for an autumn evening. Don't worry if you're not star material. You'll find there are quite enough amateur prima donnas to go round. Companies are always desperate for scene painters, wardrobe ladies, general helpers.

4. **Help out** Charity work will give you a sense of self worth and open your eyes to just how lucky you are. Most charities will be grateful for your input on any level from humble flag-selling to hands-on work. Choose your charity carefully though. Helping out is hard work and your heart needs to be in it if you're to be any use at all. If you are easily depressed then clearly being at the end of a Samaritan's telephone is not for you. If you like company then any of the charity shops will be glad of a few hours of your time and bring you in contact with the general public. There's meals-on-wheels, hospital visiting, riding for the disabled, work with the old, the young or the handicapped. If you're a good organiser you might get together a jumble or car-boot sale. If you're a good talker with business contacts consider fund-raising on a larger scale. Naturally you wouldn't go into voluntary work with an eye to the main chance but keep in mind that it can also lead on to full-time employment.

5. **Get involved** Chose a political party or a cause, anything from Greenpeace to local citizens action groups. Go to rallies/meetings. Make your voice heard. Don't think you can't make a difference: you *can*.

6. **Open up** If the kids have gone and the house feels so huge and empty that you're seriously thinking of buying a smaller place, think again. Selling the accumulated treasures of a lifetime can be very depressing. You'll also find that most of the furniture which fits into your present rooms will be too big in a more modest dwelling so that even the things you've decided to keep may have to go. If you move from the area you may lose touch with what friends you do have.

A more positive step would be to open the house up. If you're missing your children why not take in a homesick student? If your *raison d'etre* for the last twenty years has been looking after your family here's your chance to use those nurturing skills *and* make a little money. Local authorities, universities, and polytechnics are desperate for good accommodation at reasonable rates. Contact them if you think taking in a lodger is an option. You'll be making meals anyway, so what's one more mouth to feed? You'll have the spare room there, probably already set up for studying, so you won't even have to buy any furniture. If you're worried about the holidays, remember term-times coincide more or less nationwide, so when your student moves out, the room will be there for your children to move back in should they so wish.

7. **Be creative** If you've always secretly harboured an urge to write a book or even just short stories for magazines, now's your chance to have a go. Enrol for an evening course in creative writing or join the local Writers' Circle. Who knows, you might turn out to be the new Maeve Binchey. If not it's good to get away from the dinner dishes and meet with kindred spirits once a week. Alternatively, sign up for lessons that

leave you something concrete to show off at the end of term: dressmaking, machine knitting, furniture restoration, pottery. Otherwise consider a subject that will be useful and save you money, like plumbing or car maintenance. If you take a language, plump for one that's a little more out of the ordinary than French or Spanish – Russian for instance. The world is getting smaller.

8. **Learn/teach** Go back to school, either part or full time. It will bring you into contact with all sorts of people, and it will challenge and open up your mind. If you've always wanted to study archeology or computing but are stuck in a hum-drum job, you may be able to get a grant as a mature student and take a sabbatical to study full time. If you don't want to be so drastic then you can learn something that will take you into the marketplace and help you help others. The Medau Society, the Margaret Morris Movement Centre and Extend all run part-time courses, and are particularly eager to recruit mature students to teach exercise to mature pupils. Or you could try counselling, remedial massage, beauty therapy or hairdressing, all skills which, at least, can offer you a certain amount of financial independence or, at best, lay the foundations for your own alternative business.

9. **Branch out** If you used to be the best secretary in town before you got married, think about updating your expertise. It can be hard to work up the courage to get out of the house and into the thick of things again, but bringing yourself up to date with a course or work-shop can be a great confidence booster.

If you are already in gainful employment, or there are no suitable openings in your area, ask yourself whether starting your own business might not be just what you need to break out of the rut and open up your whole life. Think of what you enjoy and do best (from word-processing to cookery) and ask yourself whether anyone would pay you for it. See what grants or set-up schemes are available locally (ask at the Citizen's Advice Bureau, the library or the DSS). Try some market research, sort out your business plan (there are lots of books on the market that will tell you how) and get on with it. Don't hang around the house. Look outwards instead of in. This is the first day of the rest of your life: make the most of it!

CHAPTER 21
SEXERCISES

There is nothing like a good sex life to bring roses to the cheeks and a sparkle to the eye. And there is no good reason why sex should cease with age. If the pressures of raising a family have made this perfectly natural activity less than a priority in your life style over the past few years, then 50-plus is the perfect time to re-discover the joys of sex.

Women of a certain age, released from the possibility of unwanted pregnancy, the restrictions of 'the curse' and the risks (however small) of being on the pill can, perhaps for the first time in their lives, lie back and make the most of love-making.

There is no doubt that a well-toned body will give you more confidence and sex appeal – one more good reason to follow the routine at the beginning of the book. But, as an added bonus, here are a few 'sport specific' exercises that will add an extra zest to your sex life.

THE CAT

A Yoga-based stretch, this is wonderful for general mobility and keeping the spine from seizing up. The fluid movement is also very comforting if you suffer from dysmenorrhoea (painful periods).

Begin on hands and knees, hands under the points of the shoulders, knees hip-width apart, stomach pulled in to prevent the back from sagging. Imagine that aforementioned invisible piece of string is now attached to the centre of your back at waist level, and that someone in the skylight is hauling it up so that your spine arches upwards towards the ceiling. Allow the head to drop forward between the arms, keeping the neck relaxed. To make the most of the stretch, push the pelvis forward, pressing it towards your face. Hold for a slow count of four.

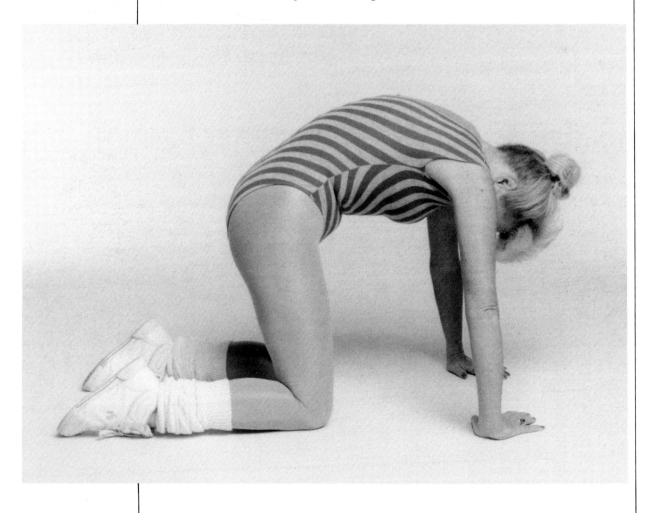

Now relax down to a position where the back is flat and parallel to the floor. Depending on the length of your arms, you may need to bend the elbows slightly. Raise your head so that you are looking directly down. If you're doing it right, there will be a straight line from the crown of the head to the tailbone. Keep your stomach pulled in and up against the spine for support. Hold again for a slow count of four.

If you have problems with your back, simply repeat these two movements twice more, holding for four each time.

If you have no problems with your back, you can go on to position three, which is to drop the back down into an arch, pushing your bottom up and raising your head up and back as though trying to reach the tailbone with the crown of the head. If you feel any pressure in the back of the neck or the lower back, come back to the flat-back position. If everything feels all right, hold this position for a count of four, and, moving back through the neutral position, go through the three positions three more times.

Think of the way a cat moves. Slinky. Sensual. Think too of a cat's reputation for going 'out on the tiles'. Perform this stretch as you feel a cat would do to make you feel super sexy. It's the perfect one to do just before you get into bed.

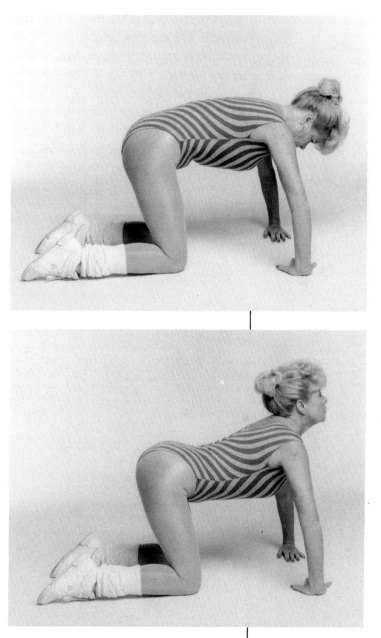

*H*IP HIP HOORAY

This exercise will gently loosen up the inside thighs and the hip joints.

Sit up straight with shoulders relaxed and chin parallel to the floor. Form the legs into a diamond. Don't bring the heels too close to the behind.

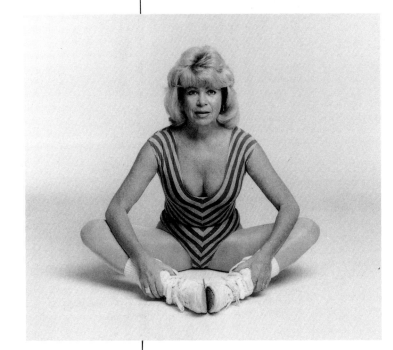

Now, with arms resting lightly on the knees, hands cupped loosely round the ankles, raise the body up and forward like the figurehead on a ship. Keeping the back straight, press the breastbone down a couple of inches towards the well between your legs. Don't round the shoulders or drop the head forward.

Hold this position for two slow counts of eight, breathing regularly and evenly, then ease yourself upright, stretch the legs out in front and shake out any tension.

Note: *never* try to loosen up the inside thigh by using force to press the knees down towards the floor. This is a delicate area of your anatomy and needs to be treated with respect. Remember, everything comes to him who waits. If your inside thighs are tight, it will take a little time to ease them out.

V FOR VICTORY

Having done that, it's time to strengthen up the inside thigh muscles.

Lie flat on your back. Arms by your sides, neck and shoulders relaxed.

Curl your knees into your chest and then stretch your legs straight up in the air. Be careful not to let them fall forwards. Bring your heels together. Flex your toes and turn them out to the sides.

Now drop your legs outwards towards the floor. Gently. Control the movement. When they've gone as far as they can go, reverse the movement by pushing in and up with the inside thigh. Not so easy. Breathe in as the legs open, out as you close them. Make sure your back doesn't arch. Keep the back of the waist pressed firmly into the floor.

Repeat eight times.

Now bring the toes together and the heels apart for a count of eight.

Finish by hugging the knees into the chest for a few moments before you go on to the next exercise.

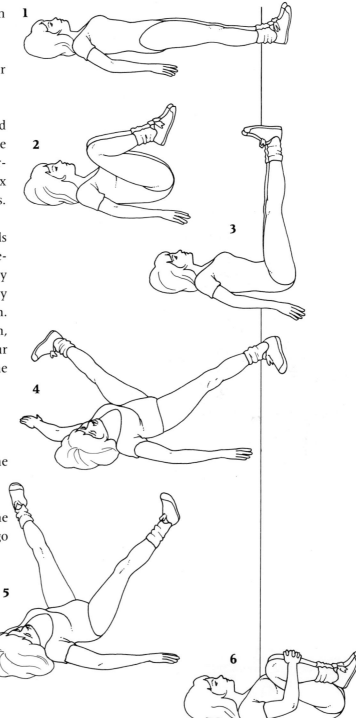

INTERNALS

For superior sex you need good, strong interior muscles as well. The following will tone up the vaginal muscles and strengthen the pelvic floor.

Lie flat, arms by your sides, knees and feet hip-width apart, knees bent up towards the ceiling, feet flat on the floor.

Now push down with your lower arms and raise your back off the floor, taking the weight on your shoulders rather than on your neck. Try not to arch your back. If you tilt your pubic bone up towards the ceiling, it should ease the hollow out behind your waist. Ideally, you should make a long, straight line from shoulder to knee. Concentrate on everything you can feel inside your pelvic girdle.

Tighten up your back passage, then your front passage and finally, try to pull the pelvic floor up towards the top of your head. Hold the position – but *not* your breath – for a moment, then relax.

Now try more control. Tighten in and up gradually for a count of four, hold for four and relax for four.

If you repeat this exercise three or four times a day, not only should you soon be able to tighten and release your vaginal and pelvic floor muscles at will, you won't 'leak' when you cough or sneeze and you'll be much more comfortable doing aerobics – which some women avoid because of stress incontinence brought on by the weakening of the pelvic floor during pregnancy and childbirth.

Sometimes it's difficult to locate your internals. You can't see them, of course, you have to rely on your sense of feel. Here's how to do it:

Next time you 'spend a penny', try to stop in mid-flow. The muscles you use to perform this feat are the ones we're talking about. When you know what it feels like to contract and relax them in one situation, you can adapt that feeling to whatever situation springs to mind!

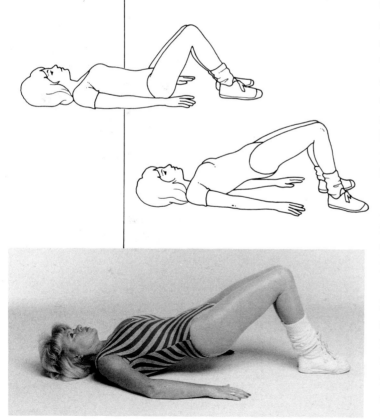

Doing the exercise in the position illustrated is perhaps the most effective method, since the law of gravity will be assisting you to pull in and up. However, you can perform the tightening and releasing standing up too. And, since no one can see you doing it, you can give your 'internals' a work-out any time, any place, anywhere.

*B*ELLY DANCERS

Stand straight, knees and feet hip width apart, toes turned out slightly for balance. Bend the knees a fraction, tuck the stomach in. Raise the arms to shoulder height at the side and, keeping the top half of the body steady but relaxed, rotate the lower half in a big circle to the right. Do eight slowly, sensuously. Enjoy it. Centre the pelvis and repeat the process, making eight big circles to the left.

This movement facilitates lots of sexual conjugations and focuses the mind on the area in question. Try it just before you slip between the sheets.

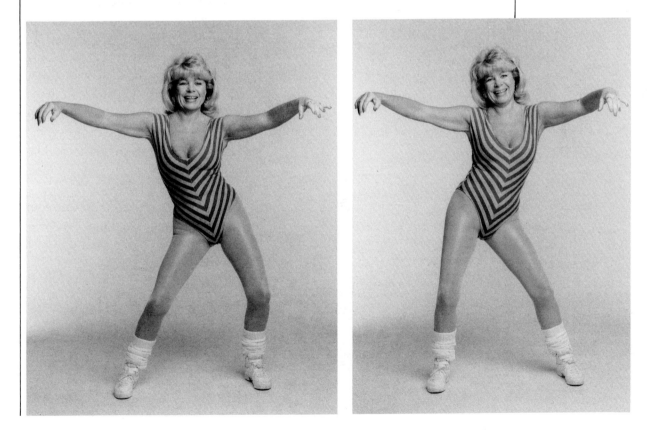

CHAPTER 22
NEW LIFE RESOLUTIONS

1. Start an exercise programme, and stick to it. Don't work in splurges: little and often is the recipe for success.

2. Cut as much fat as possible out of your diet. Drink in moderation, and give up cigarettes.

3. Learn to relax, you know it makes sense.

4. Pace yourself. Take a mini break when you need it, even if it's only a day by the sea.

5. Read a book every month, something you normally *wouldn't* read. Watch a TV programme you normally wouldn't watch. Keep informed.

6. Get involved. Join something – anything – which brings you in contact with other people.

7. Set goals. Learn one new skill every year – swimming, ski-ing, word-processing, something that will challenge you and give you a sense of achievement.

8. Call a friend or write a letter every week.

9. Don't be afraid to treat yourself well. You deserve it, don't you?

10. Be positive. Why say 'No' if you can say 'Yes'?

Write these resolutions out and put them where you'll see them often during the day. Then they'll become second nature to you.

FURTHER READING

Arpel, Adrien, *How to Look 10 Years Younger*, Warner Books Inc, New York

Bates, W.H., MD, *Better Eyesight Without Glasses*, Mayflower

Binney, Ruth (Editor) and Wright, H. Beric, MB, FRCS, MFOM (Consultant Editor), *The Complete Manual of Fitness and Well-Being*, Macdonald

Cannon, Geoffrey, *Dieting Makes You Fat*, Century

Cooper, Kenneth H. MD, MPH, *Aerobics*, Bantam Books

Grant, Doris and Joice, Jean, *Food Combining for Health*, Thorsons

Hanssen, Maurice, *E for Additives*, Thorsons

Hoare, Sophy, *Yoga*, Macdonald Educational

Jackson, Carole, *Colour Me Beautiful*, Piatkus Books

Jackson, Carole, *Colour Me Beautiful Make-up Book*, Piatkus Books

Kenton, Leslie, *The Joy of Beauty*, Century

Kenton, Leslie and Susannah, *Raw Energy Recipes*, Century

Klein, Dr Gloria, *Face Up*, Orbis

Madders, Jane, *Stress and Relaxation*, Macdonald Optima

Marshall, Lyn, in consultation with the BBC Continuing Educational Advisory Council, *Lyn Marshall's Everyday Yoga*, BBC Books

Maxwell-Hudson, Claire, *The Complete Book of Massage*, Dorling Kindersley

Mitchell, Laura and Dale, Barbara, *Simple Movement*, John Murray

Ryman, Danielle, *The Aromatherapy Handbook*, Century

Sharpe, Robert, *Thrive on Stress*, Souvenir Press

Spillane, Mary, *The Complete Style Guide*, Piatkus Books

Trimmer, Dr Eric, *The 10-Day Relaxation Plan*, Piatkus Books

von Furstenberg, Ira, *Young at Any Age*, Weidenfeld and Nicolson

Welch, Raquel, *The Raquel Welch Total Beauty and Fitness Programme*, Macmillan

Wright, Celia, *The Wright Diet*, Grafton

Tapes

Relaxatape by Samantha Lee
Available from:
Samantha Lee's Shape-up Studio
74 Bon Accord Street
Aberdeen
AB1 2EJ

Relaxation Tapes from New World
    Cassettes
Paradise Farm
Westhall
Halesworth
Suffolk
IP19 8RH

Video

Eva Fraser's Facial Workout, Virgin

HANDY ADDRESSES

The Alexander Technique
20 London House
266 Fulham Road
London
SW10 9EL
Tel. 071 351 0828

The Backstore
330 King Street
Hammersmith
London
W6 0RR
Tel. 081 741 5022

Carita House
Stapeley
Nantwich
Cheshire
CW5 7LJ
Tel. 0270 627722

Champneys
Wigginton
Tring
Herts
HP23 6HY
Tel. 0442 873155

Colour Me Beautiful
66 Abbey Business Centre
Ingate Place
London
SW8 3NS
Tel. 071 627 5211

Extend
3 The Boulevard
Shellingham
Norfolk
NR26 8LJ
Tel. 0263 822479

The Feldenkrais Association UK
PO Box 1207
Hove
East Essex
BN3 2GG
Tel. 081 549 9583

The Flotation Tank Association
(Sarah Denning/Ron Kemney, Co-Presidents)
South London Natural Health Centre
Tel. 081 728 8817

Great Company Dining Club
59 Rupert Street
London
W1V 7HN
Tel. 071 287 4540

Green Farm
Natural Health Products
Burwash Common
East Sussex
TN19 7LX
Tel. 0435 882482

House of Colour
19 Chalcot Road
London
NW1 8LL
Tel. 071 722 1984

London Clothesline Ltd
PO Box 93
London
SE23 3XS
Tel. 081 291 4375/4093/3049

Claire Maxwell-Hudson School of Massage
87 Dartmouth Road
Willesden Green
London
NW2 4ER
Tel. 081 450 6494

Mayfair Pharmacy
108 Mount Street
London
W1Y 5HE
Tel. 071 499 2597

The Medau Society
8b Robson House
East Street
Epsom
Surrey
KT17 1HH
Tel. 03727 29056

Margaret Morris Movement Centre
(Jim Hastie, Administrator and Trainer)
Head Office
Suite 3/4
39 Hope Street
Glasgow
G2 6AG
Tel. 0436 810215

Joan Price's Face Place
33 Cadogan Street
Chelsea
London
SW3 2PP
Tel. 071 589 9062

Danielle Ryman Aromatherapy
Room 101
Park Lane Hotel
Piccadilly
London
N1
Tel. 071 499 6321

The Sanctuary
11–12 Floral Street
Covent Garden
London
WC2E 9DH
Tel. 071 240 9635

Solitaire Travel Ltd
8 Melbourne Street
Royston
Herts
SG8 7BZ
Tel. 0763 249344

Stobo Castle Health Spa
Stobo
Near Peebles
Peeblesshire
EH45 8NY
Tel. 07216 249

Wardrobe
3 Grosvenor Street
London
W1
Tel. 071 629 7044

and

17 Chiltern Street
London
W1
Tel. 071 935 4086

BIBLIOGRAPHY

Arpel, Adrien, *How to Look 10 Years Younger*, Warner Books Inc, New York, 1980

Cisar, Craig J. PhD and Kravitz, Len, MA, 'Turning Back Time: Exercise and Aging', *Idea Today*, January 1991, Volume 9, Number 1

Donovan, Grant, BPE (Hons), Gianoli, Peter, BPE, Dip Ed, McNamara, Jane, BPE, Dip Ed, AIWA. *Exercise, Stop, Danger*, Wellness Australia Pty Ltd, 1989

Fonda, Jane, *Jane Fonda's Workout Book*, Allen Lane, 1982

Glass, Justine, *Eat and Stay Young*, Icon, 1961

Gillie, Oliver, Haddon, Celia, and Mercer, Derrik, (Editors), *The Sunday Times New Book of Body Maintenance*, Peerage, 1985

Jackson, Carole, *Colour Me Beautiful*, Piatkus, 1983

Klein, Dr Gloria, *Face Up*, Orbis, 1984

Kenton, Leslie, *The Joy of Beauty*, Century, 1983

Madders, Jane, *Stress and Relaxation*, MacDonald Optima, 1979

Mitchell, Laura, and Dale, Barbara, *Simple Movement*, John Murray, 1980

Newton-Dunn, Esme, *The Bodywork Book*, Collins Willow, 1982

Robbins, Tony, *Personal Power – A 30-Day Programme for Unlimited Success*, Guthy-Renker Corporation, 1989

Sharpe, Robert, *Thrive on Stress*, Souvenir Press, 1985

van der Gelder, Naneene, (Editor), *Aerobic Dance Exercise Instructor Manual*, IDEA Foundation, 1987